THE HIDDEN DRUG

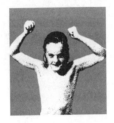

DIETARY PHOSPHATE

*Cause of Behaviour Problems, Learning Difficulties
and Juvenile Delinquency*

Hertha Hafer

THE HIDDEN DRUG

DIETARY PHOSPHATE

*Cause of Behaviour Problems, Learning Difficulties
and Juvenile Delinquency*

This book is a translation of the sixth revised edition of
"Die heimliche Droge Nahrungsphosphat, Ursache für Verhaltensstörungen,
Schulversagen und Jugendkriminalität", published in 1998 by
Hüthig Verlagsgemeinschaft, Decker & Müller GmbH,
Heidelberg in Germany.

Translated by
Jane Donlin

Edited by
Richard Jeffreys

National Library of Australia Cataloguing-in-Publication data:

Hafer, Hertha
[Die heimliche Droge Nahrungsphosphat, Ursache für Verhaltensstörungen, Schulversagen und Jugendkriminalität.]
English: The Hidden Drug – Dietary Phosphate: Cause of Behaviour Problems, Learning Difficulties and Juvenile Delinquency.

Bibliography

ISBN 0 646 40644 2.

1. Naturopathy. 2. Attention-deficit-disordered children.
3. Phosphates. 4. Food – Physiological effect.
I. Donlin, Jane. II. Jeffreys, Richard. III. Title.

612.3926

© *German edition: Georg Thieme Verlag*

© *English translation: Jane Donlin, 2001*

Enquiries concerning copyright should be directed to:
PHOSADD Australia, 112 Amethyst Crescent, Armadale 6112, Western Australia, www.phosadd.com

Cover design and Typesetting (in the New Baskerville): YPS Peter Neumann, Hamburg Germany

TRANSLATOR'S PREFACE

I specifically wish to thank:

Jillian Betts, John Dawson,
Richard Jeffreys, Dr Ernst De Jong
and Suzanne Doorey

who so generously gave of their time
and support in assisting with
this translation.

Jane Donlin

In this book Hertha Hafer studies the subject of phosphate in food and its link to Attention Deficit Disorder (ADD), allergies and other illnesses. In German the term "Attention Deficit Disorder" is not used; instead the terms "Minimal Cerebral Dysfunction" (MCD) or "Hyperkinetic Syndrome" (HKS) are used to describe the disorder.

Hertha Hafer questions whether Attention Deficit Disorder adequately describes the syndrome, because the attention deficit is only one aspect of the entire affliction. She explains: "The term 'Attention Deficit Disorder' is too restrictive and inaccurate. Cerebral dysfunction affects not only the attention span but also the entire metabolic system. Our research has revealed that a whole complex of allergies (asthma, hay fever, etc.) and skin disorders (especially neuro-dermatitis) stems from these food influences. Attention Deficit Disorder is therefore much too narrow as a term to describe the conditions we are discussing."

However, in this translation we have used the term Attention Deficit Disorder in place of the German 'Minimal Cerebral Dysfunction' because – despite Hertha Hafer's understandable concerns about its adequacy – it is the term by which the disorder is generally known in most of the English-speaking world.

It very soon became evident to our family that our son had to keep to the basic, natural foods that Hertha Hafer so highly recommends. He lost his sense of well-being whenever he consumed processed foods, soft drinks, etc. In recognising the significance of this, we are exceptionally grateful to Hertha Hafer for her research work.

Jane Donlin

Contents

INTRODUCTION TO THE SIXTH REVISED EDITION

Twenty years ago, when I first asked criminologist Professor Armand Mergen to give his opinion on this text, I would not have even dreamt that the book would be reprinted more than five times. Sincere thanks are due to Professor Mergen, who initially made its publication possible.

Today I can confidently declare not only that my findings have been verified over time but that we have also gained immense insight into the problem of phosphate-sensitivity. It is no longer a question of 10 – 20 per cent of males being affected by the syndrome but of the entire population reacting in one way or another to excessive or inadvisable consumption of certain foods. Clearly, as the Second World War demonstrated, the human organism can cope more easily with malnutrition than with an overindulgence in food that is harmful to its well-being.

Our soils are continuously being depleted of their natural nutrients by repeated cultivation of the same piece of land. However, Liebig (1803 – 73) discovered that simple mineral salts could replace the essential nutrients and mass-production of food became practicable. This discovery made it possible to feed the growing industrial population, which brought to an end years of starvation in famine-stricken Europe. Then the transport system developed and was refined; steamships and the railway system were utilised to import exotic fruit and vegetables. A world economy developed, resulting in a situation where whatever any country produced could be distributed and consumed world-wide.

The above is something of an oversimplification but it does explain why today we eat such a wide range of foods, without being concerned about where they are produced. We have forgotten how to select food that is good for our health. And as no one teaches us how to do this and many people would feel deprived if unable to eat whatever they like, it is very difficult – if not impossible – to convince people that we have to be very selective in our choice of foods if we want to live a 'healthy' life. ´

Individuals who are affected by the harmful substances in certain foods react in very different ways; for example, they affect the brain function of those with behaviour problems; people with sensitive skin develop neuro-dermatitis; and those who have asthma or other allergies react with immuno-deficiency problems. Clearly, the food we eat influences the way our immune system works. Our individual genetic inheritance determines how and to what extent the symptoms manifest themselves.

Not long ago we received a letter from Switzerland. The unfortunate child concerned suffered from just about every imaginable symptom of food poisoning. I have been able to observe that when a sensitive person continues to consume food that is harmful to him, he will suffer all his life from the symptoms. Studies that have recently been carried out in Sweden have confirmed these observations (cf. Chapter 2.9).

Recent reports from Switzerland, Australia, Sweden, the USA and Germany are so remarkably consistent that they too can be taken as further evidence.

Nutritional specialists from Sweden and Norway attended a congress at the Vidar Clinic in Järna, Sweden, in March 1997. On this occasion Dr Osika, Head of the Vidar Clinic, reported that they had achieved excellent results with my diet. Patients now routinely receive my diet (Inquiries to: S 153 31, Vidar Clinic, Järna/Sweden).

We are hopeful that further research will nurture the seed which has now taken root in sound scientific soil and thus prevent this malady of today's civilisation from claiming ever-increasing numbers of victims.

Hertha Hafe, Mainz, September 1997

PREFACE TO THE FIFTH EDITION

Our knowledge of the effects of phosphate on humans has increased since the publication of the Fourth Edition of this book. It is therefore all the more incomprehensible that the 'Phosphate-League' which we founded no longer investigates the full spectrum of symptoms. Instead it has become the 'Research Study Group on the Hyperactive Child', concerning itself with one symptom only. We deeply regret this, especially as there is no obvious reason for it.

The affliction of our civilisation is a toxicity caused by a single substance, which affects one specific type of enzyme, an affliction which makes its presence felt everywhere where phosphate-toxicity gives rise to symptoms. Recently, a whole range of other substances – for example preservatives, stabilisers and colouring agents – has been blamed for causing ADD but as yet no conclusive evidence has been found to support such claims.

When it became known that phosphate in cleaning products had a damaging effect on natural eco-systems, environmentally concerned citizens very quickly instigated successful programs to protect plants, waterways, marine life and so on. In contrast, to date it has not been possible to generate a similar level of community concern about the terrible damage being done to the well-being of our children.

This book aims to present explanations of the causes and effects of phosphate sensitivity based primarily on our experiences and observations, as we do not have access to a research facility to conduct a clinical trial with which to prove statistically our now well-supported hypotheses.

I again call upon the medical profession, as I have done so many times in the past, to duplicate the experiments described in this book and then to explain their observations scientifically.

Researchers need to investigate these findings seriously for the sake of the victims' health. The work is urgent as a single dose of approximately 125mg phosphorus, which is equivalent to 75mg phosphate (PO_4), can lead to a relapse.

When we are speaking of phosphate (PO_4), we will always be referring to PO_4, irrespective of the source of phosphoric acid.

The majority of people are not phosphate-sensitive; they can eat whatever they like. Those who are sensitive, however, need to understand their sensitivity and especially to realise that for the time being there is no possibility of overcoming it or healing it through therapy.

The danger for our sensitive children is especially the corner shop where they can buy soft drinks, sausages, sweets and other general junk-food, causing them to relapse into their previous condition.

We aim to inform as many phosphate-sensitive people as possible and to provide them with the resources to help themselves.

Montreux, February 1990

Hertha Hafer

INTRODUCTION

In January 1988 Swiss Professor Mark R. Bachmann posed the question: "Why have the oft recurring outbursts of criticism of food and food technology led to so little constructive debate between consumers on the one hand and food manufacturers on the other?" He was writing under the heading of chemistry in a renowned trade journal for Science, Technology and Economics. In his presentation he called upon consumers and opinion-makers to stick to the facts (instead of posturing) and to replace confrontation with rigorous analysis. He also cautioned his own colleagues against falling into the trap of thinking that they had all the answers.

"In the field of nutrition," Bachmann wrote, "as in all fields, we are continually gaining more knowledge. The main source of knowledge is research. However, time and again discoveries are made outside the established research centres. More discerning observers can gain knowledge and perceive connections, either incidentally or after being involved with a problem for a long time. If such a discovery is made, two things can happen; either the discovery is rejected out of hand or it is analysed scientifically and then confirmed or rejected. In the field of nutrition there are examples of both reactions. Usually, however, such a discovery encounters immediate rejection when it runs counter to established doctrines or opposes the interests of the food industry. This is regrettable; after all, it has been known since Galileo Galilei that even established doctrines can sometimes be wrong".

Bachmann presented an example of this (of particular interest to the reader of this book) when he talked of the problem of phosphate in food. He described it "as causing a certain form of 'psycho-somatic syndrome' in children, the so-called Attention Deficit Disorder (ADD) and/or Attention Deficit Hyperactivity Disorder (ADHD)". To the food expert such a claim appears at first glance to be absurd. He knows that phosphate participates in vital energy conversions in all living organisms, including humans, and that phosphate is an essential element of bone matter.

Bachmann explained that food experts consider phosphate a desirable component of food and that humans consume considerable amounts daily. In childhood many of us were given 'tonics' by the spoonful for "the positive effect they had on certain phospholipids[1] of the brain and its ability to learn". Thus we can see very clearly why food experts find the title 'The Hidden Drug – Dietary Phosphate' incomprehensible. Bachmann felt that these experts should investigate the topic thoroughly, rather than simply dismissing it as apparent provocation. Moreover, Bachmann made an observation that particularly applies to the author of this book. He said: "Someone who has personal experience of Attention Deficit Disorder is more likely to study closely whether phosphate is a drug and to ascertain whether the allegation is genuine."

So it was fortuitous that Hertha Hafer, a research pharmacist of many years' experience and her husband, a chemist working for a well-known pharmaceutical company, had a hyperactive son. Their combined scientific knowledge and experience predisposed them to make observations and draw conclusions more accurately than most parents. One result was that under certain specific conditions they noticed that their maladjusted son could behave completely 'normally'; he was unusually responsive and sociable. These events are comprehensively described in this book. A further advantage that these parents had was access to the relevant English-language literature. Thus they knew that the American doctor Ben Feingold had observed back in 1972 in the USA how altering the diet of children changed their behaviour.

Hertha Hafer ascertained, whilst observing her son and other

1: *A phosphorylated lipid which is a major component of cell membranes.*

afflicted children in her neighbourhood, that they became responsive, friendly companions when they were consistently given low-
phosphate food. She became convinced that a daily excess of
phosphate in food was responsible for behaviour problems.

Bachmann posed the logical question: "Is there more phosphate in food today than in the past?" He referred to the German
Health Department which recommends a daily intake of 750mg
phosphorus per adult. Feldheim calculated the actual intake to be
1570mg per adult per day, which is more than double the recommended amount. "Undoubtedly the more industrially prepared
foods we consume, the greater is our intake of phosphate. Phosphate
has been generally considered harmless, which has led the food
industry to use it increasingly as an additive. The excellent properties
of phosphate when used in buffer solutions, emulsifiers, stabilisers,
thickeners, anti-oxidants, etc. have resulted in its being regarded as a
versatile and highly effective additive. The meat industry uses phosphate, as mineral salts, in sausages and other ham and bologna style
coldcuts. Phosphate is also found in cheese spreads and is used as an
emulsifier in soups, sauces, creams and chocolates. It occurs in food
as a flour improver, a flow conditioner in bulk goods, an aerator and
as a component of modified starch".

Petra Kühne, a food scientist working in Frankfurt, also
pointed out the discrepancy between the recommended amount of
phosphorus and the actual intake. She did this specifically for children and differentiated between girls and boys as well as different age
groups:

RECOMMENDED INTAKE OF PHOSPHORUS *mg per day*			ACTUAL INTAKE OF PHOSPHORUS *mg per day*	
Age in Years	Males	Females	Males	Females
4 – 6	700	700	1021	829
7 – 9	800	800	1147	936
10 – 12	1000	900	1270	1043

| 13 – 14 | 1000 | 1000 | 1365 | 1112 |
| 15 – 18 | 900 | 800 | 1571 | 1249 |

Petra Kühne[2] stressed the fact that we should not just consider the one element (phosphorus) because there is a relationship between phosphorus and calcium. "If 800mg phosphorus is recommended daily, 800mg calcium should also be recommended daily, i.e. phosphorus and calcium should be consumed in a 1:1 ratio. This quantity of calcium, however, is rarely consumed. The greater intake of phosphorus changes the phosphorus-calcium ratio and brings about an imbalance".

Media reports have made us aware of the many children who obviously cannot tolerate the oversupply of phosphate, of how much they and their parents suffer from their hyperactivity and of how teachers and fellow students – just to mention those in their immediate environment – experience the 'fidget' in their class. Gerd Biermann believed that children with the hyperactive syndrome were 'problem children'. He said, "Their psychomotor restlessness and their hyperactivity, which develops into aggression, constantly cause conflict with those who endeavour to adjust and integrate them into their environment".

In the summer of 1987 a Swiss television station reported on this phenomenon. After the broadcast, about 20,000 interested families, whose children were suffering from the symptoms described, made inquiries about the program. This only confirms what we have been observing for many years in Germany, in the rest of Europe and also in the USA; there are more and more children suffering from behaviour difficulties, ever more despairing parents and helpless educators.

2: Petra Kühne: Reform Rundschau, 2/1987

On 26 October 1987 Dr Walter Eichlseder, a paediatrician from Munich, reported the results of an investigation involving 5,000 children. The children were interviewed using the 'Conners-questionnaire'. The results revealed that twenty per cent of primary school children were hyperactive and six per cent of secondary school children. The percentage in the Senior High Schools was smaller. Unfortunately the investigation did not include schools for children with special needs. Eichlseder found there were always more boys than girls affected.

On 12 May 1988 the 'Neuss-Grevenbroicher Newspaper' published an article about a course organised by the Youth Welfare Office of the township of Neuss. A hundred educators – primary school teachers, trained youth workers and other associated workers – attended the course. At that gathering Hans Jürgen Heubach from Düsseldorf, a psychiatrist specialising in adolescent problems, lectured on the ADD-syndrome (medical name for the phenomenon 'hyperactive children'). This is also evidence of how topical the subject had become. On that occasion the lecturer stated that the participation of educators was "crucial", because the "disorder has first to be recognised as such". He pointed out that it first becomes apparent in the play misdemeanours of small children and then goes on to manifest itself in the form of learning difficulties in children of school age.

Heubach also mentioned the frequent reports in the media about phosphate in food, which supposedly is responsible for causing aggression in children. "Investigations confirm that in twenty-five to thirty per cent of children diagnosed with ADD, the low-phosphate diet has brought about a marked improvement". A well-known office for child and adolescent psychiatry and psychotherapy run by Dr Richard Schydlo and Dr Jürgen Heubach in Düsseldorf provided these results. They had been investigating the problem for a long time.

Dr Heubach said at the end of his lecture in Neuss that there was still controversy over whether or not diet could eliminate the actual causes of behaviour problems. Hertha Hafer had not claimed this; she had merely written down her personal observations and experiences, which were first published in 1978 under the title: 'Phosphate in Food as a Cause of Behaviour Difficulties and Juvenile Delinquency'. She had expected that this would lead to a serious investigation of her observations according to standard scientific practice.

Since that time Hertha Hafer's book has achieved a large circulation, even outside Germany: In 1984 it was published in French and in 1990 it was translated into Italian. Numerous support groups for parents emerged in Germany as well as abroad (this organisation of parents is known as the Research Study Group for the Hyperactive Child, formerly called the Phosphate League and the Swiss Phosphate League). These groups have tested Hertha Hafer's findings and have confirmed that the low-phosphate diet is practical and helpful and, on the basis of that experience, have sought to inform the general public.

There were, however, especially among scientists, many opponents of the Hafer theory. Some dismissed Hertha Hafer's work as unscientific and warned against the use of the recommended diet. For example Prof F Bläker and Prof Dr J Martinius classified the diet as "precarious".

According to Hafer the evidence on which Profs Bläker and Martinius relied and which the scientific establishment has used and still uses today, derives from a single piece of work from the time when low-phosphate diet was first discussed more than ten years ago. Consequently Hertha Hafer has accused politicians and the research establishment of negligence.

The majority of parents with afflicted children, however, recognises the value of the diet and derives very valuable help from it. Parents have no hesitation in confirming that Hertha Hafer's observations are consistent with their own. Consequently there are families who have been eating low-phosphate food for years and have shown no pathological symptoms that can be attributed to the diet; their doctors have confirmed this during regular medical check-ups.

Visitors attending the support groups observed on the one hand the despair of parents because doctors and therapists were unable to help their children and, on the other, relief and gratitude when the Hafer diet brought rapid and enduring improvement. Paediatricians, psychologists and therapists who had previously stated, "There is no scientific proof", listened attentively to parents who reported on their experiences with the diet.

There certainly are scientific findings that support Hertha Hafer's thesis. Thus H Schmidt-Gayk and W Hiltzler as well as M Kohlmann wrote: "Only a few investigations are recorded of the amount of phosphorus that each person requires. Presumably the reason for this is that there is an ample supply of phosphorus in food and the organism can adjust to different quantities as long as it does not fall below a certain level. This implies that the supply of phosphorus is sufficient when the supply of other components in food, for example protein, is adequate. A somewhat larger study involving twenty-one people demonstrated that the amount of phosphorus that each person required was approximately 0.88g per 70kg body weight (approx. 12.6mg per kg). Elsewhere Nordin and Smith stated that the amount of phosphorus required was 12.2mg per kg. These quantities correspond with the recommendations of the German Association for Nutrition. On the other hand, these values should not be seen as an absolute lower limit because more recent studies of healthy adults found that the body was able to compensate for an intake of 10mg per kg per day. The organism's ability to adapt over a large range and still achieve a balance lies in the kidney's ability to suppress phosphorus excretion into the urine. To conserve phosphorus, the kidneys excrete minimal quantities when the serum-phosphorus falls below a certain level. An insufficient supply of phosphorus evidently results in this hypo-phosphate condition and is not the result of a phosphorus imbalance. To prevent a hypo-phosphate condition, the minimum recommended amount of phosphorus must be consumed in the diet".

The authors from the University of Heidelberg even confirmed Hertha Hafer's suspicions that today's oversupply of phosphate
in food causes illnesses in all age groups − with enormously
increasing frequency. They suggested that a phosphate intake, which
is excessive in relation to the calcium intake, is responsible for the
development of osteoporosis.

The staff at some institutions proceeded according to precise
methods. In 1987 the Marl State Hospital gave twenty-two hyperactive
children low-phosphate food. It became unnecessary after a few days
to administer additional doses of psycho-pharmaceutical drugs. "In
twenty-one children a significant improvement in behaviour could be
observed". Only one child, who had brain damage, barely responded
to the change of diet. On the twenty-ninth day the children received
a normal breakfast. According to Ursula Klemm, paediatrician,
twenty minutes later they were once again 'screaming and fighting'
(DNÄ, 22 April 1987).

A statement issued by two official medical organisations
revealed that the London Hospital for Sick Children had undertaken
a larger scale experiment. They had treated children with various
disorders (migraine, hyperkinetic syndrome) with a so-called oligo-
antigenic diet. Here, controlled studies unmistakably demonstrated
that the effectiveness of this diet went far beyond that of a placebo.

Surprisingly the statement also said: "Owing to the successful
treatment of hyperactive children with the oligo-antigenic diet, the
results obtained are now being analysed seriously. Some components
of this diet correspond with low-phosphate food". It is possible
therefore that low-phosphate food has non-specific or other
independent effects besides phosphate reduction. The questions
raised, however, require verification before final judgements can be
made over dietary treatment possibilities, especially those concerning
low-phosphate food.

Unfortunately, this publication did not disclose who in Germany was going to undertake the task of 'investigating' the 'questions raised' or when. It is also not clear how it is known that these 'non-specific or other independent effects of the phosphate reduction' brought about the 'verified results'. The oligo-antigenic diet does, however, correspond in 'some components' with low-phosphate food.

Nonetheless, the declared intention is:

- to examine the differences and also the similarities between the low-phosphate food and the oligo-antigenic diet
- to research the reasons for the observed effects and
- then to make a judgement.

This is a positive move. It is to be hoped that action will soon be taken to implement these intentions!

Bachmann in his report also called for objectivity and wrote at the end of his dissertation: "The advocates of low-phosphate food talk predominantly of indications, but not of explanations of the correlation between phosphate in food and ADD. They simply assert that a massive reduction of phosphate ingestion leads to the disappearance of those symptoms associated with Attention Deficit Disorder. They further assert that when the children who are sensitive to it start consuming phosphate again, the physical and psychological disorders return. These observations do not explain the connection between phosphate and the syndrome; they do, however, reveal the absolute necessity for investigating the facts".

Bachmann ultimately demanded a scientific clarification of the problem, just as Hertha Hafer and the many afflicted people have done for more than ten years.

Wiltrud Wehner-Davin/Bernd Wehner

REVISED INTRODUCTION TO THE SIXTH EDITION

Hertha Hafer's book: The Hidden Drug – Dietary Phosphate was first published almost twenty-five years ago. It has since been reprinted six times and is to this day receiving considerable attention.

A new generation of parents is reading her book, following her advice, reporting their experiences and is grateful to Hertha Hafer. Just like the previous generation of parents did, they describe the problems they and their children encounter. They describe how their children change dramatically when they follow the diet for a few days but they also let you know how their children very quickly revert to their previous difficult behaviour when they consume food that is not permitted.

Years later parents are still telling almost identical stories. Usually they and their children have suffered for many years before they try the diet. Is it to be wondered that they ask: "How come our family doctor had no idea how to help us?"

For many years parents – non-professionals – have been experimenting with the low-phosphate diet, have been forming self-help associations, have been exchanging their stories, have been keeping discussion alive and – most importantly – have been succeeding in helping their children, whereas the experts have remained silent.

These are the reasons why Dr G Ionescu's[3] publication titled: "Abnormal levels of catecholamine concentration in the plasma of hyperactive children" is of considerable interest.

Ionescu explains why psychological intervention has little influence on the behaviour of hyperactive children. They have a metabolism significantly different to that of 'normal' children. Research in 1989/90 revealed that the blood of hyperactive children

---

3: *Ionescu, G: Der informierte Arzt; Gazette Medicale (Basel),*
  17 pp 1665-1668 (1991)

contained abnormally high levels of vital neurohormones, called catecholamines. In particular they have chronically high levels of dopamine and epinephrine. Thus it is possible to distinguish a 'true' hyperactive child from a 'normal' child: The hyperactive child has abnormally high levels of catecholamines triggered by environmental poisoning. An uncontrolled release of neurohormones affects the entire central nervous system, a condition that can be prevented. All substances that trigger dysfunction of the nervous system have to be avoided at all times (fruit juices, soft drinks, lollies, chocolate, cookies, food additives such as sodium, phosphate and other mineral salts, eggs, milk, nuts, tomato ketchup, spices).

On 4 November 1996 German television once again broadcast a program on hyperactivity. SAT 'Akte 96/45' introduced the children concerned and their doctors.

It was most incredible and disturbing to watch American boys going so wild that even a heavily built adult man was barely able to restrain them. According to American Professor Doris Rapp, tomatoes triggered this behaviour in one of the boys, a slice of white bread in the other – very ordinary foods, which the boys had eaten just before.

Psychologist Cordula Neuhaus has studied hyperactive children and their families over an extensive period of time. She believes that the attention deficit syndrome is caused by brain dysfunction. Hyperactive children suffer from an inability to filter certain stimuli and impulses, which is hereditary. Frequently the fathers suffered from the same syndrome as their children. Neuhaus described them as being fit, creative, likeable, sociable and aware but also as suffering from mood swings, anxiety, depression and drug addiction. Father and child experience similar impulsiveness, inattentiveness, an inability to concentrate; they flare-up easily and are hyperactive. They feel deeply rejected, they crave love and attention and yet they are highly critical of others.

Hertha Hafer is convinced that hyperactivity increasingly affects all age groups; it is not a problem that will eventually be outgrown.

When, because of their genetic inheritance, susceptible individuals develop a lifelong sensitivity to food, the fundamental question arises: Is it possible that the rising tide of aggression and violence in our society is the result of a dietary deficiency? American researchers have made the first attempts to answer this question. One answer reads as follows: More and more hyperactive children are becoming addicted to drugs; they are developing anti-social behaviour and turning to crime. Is all this merely a response to their daily intake of flavour-improved, preserved and emulsified bread, which so often is recommended as being highly beneficial to our health?

Wiltrud Wehner-Davin

1.0 PHOSPHATE AS A CAUSE OF BEHAVIOUR DISORDERS (ATTENTION DEFICIT DISORDER)

1.1 REPORT OF A DISCOVERY

"You, you're just naughty!" These were the words spoken by a friendly, motherly, primary school teacher to my small, chubby and pale son Michael who was standing helplessly, slightly sadly before her. I wondered what the matter was with her? He did try.

The teacher informed me that Michael did not take part in the lessons. He fidgeted, disturbed his fellow students and did not copy down words as expected from the blackboard. When she asked Michael why he did not write, he answered, "I don't feel like it!"

Nobody had realised at this stage that Michael was incapable of forming letters. The teacher quite clearly thought that Michael was a spoiled child and his parents were to be blamed and were incapable of bringing him up properly.

Michael, who was six years old at the time, had been attending primary school for six weeks. Just prior to the start of school my husband and I had adopted him but he had been living with us as 'our child' for more than four years.

In his first year of life the boy had missed out on the regular bonding with his mother. Before he came to stay with us, several different people had cared for him. At fifteen months he came to live with my husband and myself, our housekeeper (of many years standing) and her son Peter. The two boys, almost the same age, grew close like brothers. By the time Michael started school, Peter was no longer with us – his mother had married.

Michael's adjustment to his new family and his first years with us proceeded without problems. From the age of three he attended a kindergarten in which he stayed until the start of school, without having any obvious difficulties.

Prior to starting school, Michael was given a medical examination; he was found to be very light and very small of stature but nevertheless was considered mature enough to start school.

The difficulties began a few weeks after he started school. I have referred above to one of my early encounters with the school. During the following weeks there were similar occurrences.

These problems led us to seek advice from a psychologist. He examined the boy. The examination revealed that, despite a 'normal relationship' with my husband and me, Michael suffered from diffuse anxiety. The psychologist could not explain why and was not able to give us any advice.

Michael of course continued to attend school punctually and regularly. He even enjoyed going and found it interesting but his behaviour in school did not change; quite the opposite, his problems increased.

At this point I would like to put on record the fact that during the war and post-war period I had brought up a daughter under the most adverse conditions. I had been on my own and working as a professional. In due course my daughter gained her A-levels, went to University and married. Her upbringing presented no problems whatsoever. When, at the beginning of his schooling, Michael appeared to be developing into a 'problem child' I had no knowledge of behaviour difficulties in children. My husband (a chemist) and I (a pharmacist), however, were both used to scientific work and therefore found making observations and reaching conclusions easy; the following text will describe these.

We consulted a neurologist who gave Michael an intelligence test (Wechsler for children). Michael's IQ was 120 for the manual component and 126 for the verbal. After hyperventilation delta waves showed up on the EEG. The results indicated that our boy was of above average intelligence but, because of the anomaly in the EEG, he was prescribed a low dose of phenylethyl barbituric acid.

To our utmost amazement the dose of barbiturates led to a reaction opposite to that which we had expected. The boy's motor restlessness increased. As a result the doctor increased the dose. Now Michael just sat drowsily on the school bench but fidgeted continuously. This medication was stopped and Carbamazepine – a different, anti-epileptic drug – was prescribed instead. His motor restlessness increased even more. The child became scatterbrained; his condition was sufficiently serious to alarm us. We stopped giving him this medication. It has since become known that all sedatives are strictly contraindicated for children with behaviour difficulties, at least with those like Michael's.

In our despair – and we were indeed becoming more and more desperate – we sought the advice of a psychiatrist. Result: "Intelligent children are sometimes a little difficult. Give it a little time. Try Meprobamate." This medication also brought no relief.

In the years following his first year of school, Michael became increasingly incapable of keeping his belongings together and of maintaining any order or system. He always forgot something - an exercise or textbook, pens and pencils or sportswear. The mess in his bedroom was just as chaotic as that in his school bag. In his restlessness and boredom he broke pencils into small pieces and chewed them to bits; he ground erasers into crumbs and splayed his pen-nib. We had to replace the contents of his pencil case once a week.

Michael never knew what homework he had to do. He could not pay attention and lost track of a lesson after only a few minutes. He understood and remembered barely anything. At the end of each school day we telephoned the neighbours to find out what his home-work was and we tried to teach the boy ourselves. It was a miracle that he learnt anything at all in primary school.

Because Michael could not cope with the level of work, he became bored and spent all his time inventing 'new misdemeanours'. He made paper planes, threw bits of paper around, pinched the girls and pulled their hair. He ran around the classroom as he pleased, amusing his fellow students and seeking attention. He became the 'class-clown'.

The same happened in sport lessons. He fidgeted around and was incapable of doing the exercises taught. In swimming lessons Michael could not coordinate his arms and legs – he could not keep himself afloat and swim forwards at the same time. Three metres of wild thrashing about were the most he could manage.

Around this time Michael said that he felt like learning to play the piano. We were more than happy to grant his wish but it was the same as the swimming, or rather worse – he could not do it at all. His fine motor skills and coordination were impaired.

When Michael first learnt to write, his writing was unexceptional. Although his exercise books from his first school year had their peculiarities, his writing appeared acceptable. This began to change and the writing rapidly became increasingly illegible. It was impossible for Michael to keep the letters on the line, to space them evenly or to regulate their size but the form of his letters, when there was scope for a certain amount of artistic expression, was beautiful and they were very individually formed.

When one examined Michael's writing, a marked discrepancy between the activity and the person became apparent. It looked like a 'barbed wire entanglement' and yet he formed the letters like an adult.

We have since learned that it was indeed impossible for Michael to do copy writing. His teacher was in the habit of getting her students to write down text from the blackboard and then allowing them at home to make a 'clean copy' in their exercise books. Our son would sit in front of the big blackboard and begin to write a few letters in his book. He would rub them out, say he did not like his letters and that he wanted to make them more beautiful. Michael would repeat this until the paper was full of holes from all the rubbing. After hours he had written nothing or almost nothing.

When the teacher asked him why he had not written anything, she received the predictable answer: "I don't feel like it". Her response – scolding and detention. Michael did not spend just two or three hours at school (as is the custom in Germany for first grade children) but four and five.

When Michael arrived home, he had no text to make a clean copy of in his exercise book. We therefore requested this from his classmates. Soon we discovered that the boy was able to write by dictation easily and willingly. He would therefore need help to do his homework. We found a student teacher who visited us several times a week and worked with Michael. She also took him on walks, talked to him and listened to him. She had no problems with the boy; she let him work off his motor restlessness from time to time and allowed him to let off steam. A most important element of this work with the student teacher was that Michael did not have to work under the pressure of time. In class he started everything and never finished anything; he panicked under the pressure of time, whilst at home he could now tackle his tasks in peace, with pauses and without problems.

Our boy was now eight years old and his behavioural difficulties were increasing, especially at school.

The teachers, naturally, demanded more of the older child than of a six-year-old. As the boy was not able to achieve to the standard normally expected, the teachers lost patience with him. They urged us to intervene – obviously they still assumed that we were spoiling Michael.

It was by no means an easy matter for us to put up with the boy with all his problems. And we too had to agree with the teachers that Michael was an 'enfant terrible', an 'awful child'. The boy literally suffered from a destructive urge. All toys fell to pieces in his hands. His impulses also led him to destroy furniture and household items in our house, as well as to damage other people's belongings. He had shredded the coverings of our dining room chairs; the cutlery drawers had deep notches in them that Michael had carved out with a table knife. When we asked him to lay the table, he took out the knives; his next impulse was to chop, no matter where. The wooden backrest of the armchair in his room looked like a chopping block, the doors of his wardrobe as if someone had shot at them with buckshot.

Around this time a psychotherapist, who had set up practice in Mainz, attracted our attention. We sent our boy several times a week to him for treatment. In his opinion Michael's father 'dominated' him. He, the therapist, wanted to 'free' Michael from this domination. The intensive treatment lasted for a year – after which nothing had changed.

At the start of this psychotherapeutic treatment Michael also changed school. We had gained the impression that his previous teachers had reached the end of their tethers. His old primary school had been near my pharmacy; his new school was located near our home. This change of school, however, did not bring about any improvement. Quite the opposite – the 'trouble-maker' had to sit alone at the 'back of the classroom'. As a result, Michael felt that he had been sent to the bottom of the class; he felt personally rejected. His comment was: "She doesn't even put me in detention".

During the Christmas of 1969 we had a remarkable experience with Michael. On the third day of our winter holiday he came down with a very severe viral infection. For a week he was feverish – several times his temperature rose above forty degrees Celsius – but while he had such a high temperature we had a perfectly normal child. As the fever eased off and he began to recover, the behaviour difficulties returned. We had observed something like this previously when our family would occasionally quarrel, especially when we argued about Michael. Then, for three days, his behaviour would be totally unobtrusive. So it came about that Michael proved repeatedly, admittedly for short periods only, that he could be a delightful child, as I firmly believed at heart he was.

What was wrong with Michael? What was it that contorted him for extensive periods of his young life and then allowed him to be quite normal again for a short time? We lived with these questions daily.

In the summer of 1970 the education authorities of our town informed me that they were considering transferring our son to a school for children with special needs. His teacher had convinced the school authorities that Michael was unmanageable.

It didn't seem right to us to put Michael in a school for children with special needs when previous tests had revealed and demonstrated his intelligence. I therefore refused. The education authorities now threatened us with the possibility of banning Michael from compulsory education. Although we would have preferred to have left him in a normal school, so that he could live at home with us, we now tried to get him into a special therapeutic residential children's home (the cost at that time was approximately DM 1,300 monthly). We chose one in North Germany.

This special therapeutic residential children's home was a private and well-conducted institution, which accommodated children who had experienced personal problems but who otherwise had normal mental abilities. Forty-eight children lived in the home. They lived in four groups; each housed twelve boys and girls of different ages. The foster mother was either an educational psychologist or a specially trained teacher. Two psychologists, one trained as a medical practitioner, assisted the foster mother and the children. The home did not have its own school. The children instead attended ordinary schools in the area. Michael, who was nine years old at the time, repeated the third grade[4].

4: *Translator's Note: Regular promotion in schools from year to year, such as is standard practice in American and Australian schools, (continues p. 32)*

At this time (September 1970) one of our neighbours showed us an excerpt from the newspaper 'Bild-Zeitung'. Here we read that children who "were throwing things through other people's windows and who were not doing their homework" were being prescribed Ritalin in the American Hospital in Frankfurt. The treatment was a success. Methylphenidate-HCl is the generic name for Ritalin. According to the Basle parent company CIBA, it was only in the USA in those days that Ritalin was registered for the treatment of disturbed children. In Germany the company produced no information or advertising material whatsoever for this product, because of its effect as an amphetamine. They did, however, provide us with information after we had made specific inquiries. They sent us a bundle of scientific reports, published in the USA (in Europe when the Göttinger Institute of Psychiatry investigated the issue, no research had been undertaken in this direction prior to 1971).

After consulting our medical practitioner, we tentatively gave Michael a dose of 5mg Methylphenidate-HCl twice a day. Just as described in the American literature, within twenty minutes (!) our child changed totally. The restless muscle tension eased; Michael stood calm and relaxed before us. His glance steadied and he made eye contact. He kept to the subject during conversation. He listened to others without interrupting them.

The effect of Methylphenidate-HCl only lasted for four or five hours. We had but a few days left to observe Michael, as the school holidays were over and he had to return to the children's home.

We translated the information on the use and effects of the medication and gave it to the staff of the children's home, convinced that they would be interested in the continuation of this treatment. We were mistaken. The treatment was not continued and Michael was

---

is not automatic in Germany; in that country children who fail to perform adequately in any given academic grade may be held back and made to repeat the year.

again treated with psychotherapy. But this therapy met with no success. Three months after starting school in North Germany he had to be taken out of his new school, because once again his behaviour was unacceptable. After six weeks of further intensive psychotherapeutic treatment, Michael was sent back to school. In addition to other forms of treatment, he was under the care of a neurologist.

Whilst visiting Michael in early May 1971, we took him out for a meal. It was then that we noticed that Michael's motor restlessness had increased to a level that we had never experienced before. We made inquiries and were informed that the neurologist had prescribed 100mg Pyrithioxine three times a day. It was quite evident to us that the deterioration in our son's condition was due to this prescription of 100mg Pyrithioxine three times a day. Pyrithioxine is a substance which is supposed to encourage cerebral metabolism. It is also known to be contraindicated for behaviour disturbed children because it increases their motor restlessness.

My husband and I conducted a Methylphenidate-HCl experiment the next day. Michael was prescribed 100mg Pyrithioxine at the children's home; on top of that we gave him 5mg Methylphenidate-HCl. Then we drove off in the car. Twenty minutes later we had to make an emergency stop for Michael – he badly needed to go to the toilet. When he returned to the car he asked for a pillow and literally fell onto the car seat and slept quietly and totally relaxed for the next twenty minutes. After this and for the next four hours we had a normal, calm and cheerful child. During afternoon tea, we observed that Michael's feet were beginning to jig under the table. Within the next ten minutes the restlessness in his body moved upwards. His hands started to move around the table, his legs were swinging and within the next half hour all his motor restlessness had returned.

On the basis of these observations we were satisfied that the administration of Methylphenidate-HCl was the only sensible treatment to persist with.

We agreed therefore, together with the director of the home and the doctor who was treating Michael, that from then on he should be treated with Methylphenidate-HCl. The treatment started on 7 June 1971 with a daily dose of 0.35mg per kg of body weight.

For the long vacation at the end of July we fetched Michael from the children's home, so that we could take him on a holiday. During the first few days we noticed that the boy was picking his teeth after eating – he said he had bits of meat sticking in them. When I inspected his teeth I found that this child, previously totally free of dental caries, had six badly decayed baby teeth. It was clear that the medication Methylphenidate-HCl had produced sudden and devastating dental caries within six weeks. This continued all the following year and from September 1971 onwards Michael developed recurring tonsillitis as well.

These observations reminded me of earlier research work I had done. I had investigated bacteriological colonisation of the mucous membrane in the mouth and had observed that it was influenced by the metabolism. In 1956/57 we had made caries resistant rats susceptible to caries by giving them ammonia. We had planned then to follow up the test by experimenting with amphetamines, from which we expected the same results.

Here now we had an overwhelming incidence of caries in the teeth of a human being, triggered by a substance resembling amphetamine. A biochemical mechanism, similar to the result we obtained after giving ammonia to rats but much more powerful, must have changed Michael's bacterial mouth and pharynx flora rapidly and completely. Therefore, the treatment with Methylphenidate-HCl (and this applies to all amphetamines) had side effects – it changed the metabolism and caused caries in teeth and inflammation of the throat. Two years later Michael's baby teeth were profoundly decayed and, after repeated severe bouts of tonsillitis, his tonsils had to be surgically removed.

In the autumn of 1971, whilst still living in the children's home, Michael began his fourth year of school, which he completed without difficulty. He had a teacher who was strict but who liked him. She gave Michael a good report in the autumn of 1972. The junior high school (Gymnasium[5]) accepted him for enrolment.

In July 1973 we received a telephone call from the children's home; Michael, together with other children, had truanted from school for fourteen days. The children had 'organised' chains, planks and railway sleepers, had built a camp on the railway embankment and had also tied a girl to a post. This made it necessary for us to speak to the boy personally.

About this time Michael was to be admitted to hospital for the removal of his tonsils, so my husband drove to the children's home to fetch him. Michael had barely arrived home when he put a small bottle on the table, containing fourteen days' supply of Methylphenidate-HCl. He said: "I have kept these because they are so dangerous!" Then he told us that he had decided "to have a good time" and to take no more tablets. He just wanted to forget school for a while. In the home itself the truancy had not been noticed because the children had returned on time as always after school.

During this time shoplifting also occurred in department stores. I was unable to investigate the incident further (incidentally I am of the opinion that theft in department stores is a typical crime of children with these behaviour difficulties. I shall come back to this later).

From then on Michael again lived with us in Mainz. He attended the Junior High School and we continued the treatment with Methylphenidate-HCl.

In the winter of 1973/74 our doctor diagnosed Michael as having poor circulation and a blood cholesterol level that was too

---

5: *A selective school for academically gifted children*

high. We tried to reduce the dose of Methylphenidate-HCl. We only gave him a dose in the morning so that at least this would help him get through the day at school but this dosage was obviously not sufficient. The boy's behaviour worsened, especially at school. The school principal described him to his colleagues as follows:

"The boy attracted attention because of his severe behaviour disorders: an excess of inner hostility, aggression, hyperactivity, emotional instability, poor tolerance to frustration, a craving for social acknowledgment, lack of concentration, distraction, impulsiveness – yet he was highly intelligent. During the lessons the boy wrestled, caused continual disturbances, assaulted the teacher and so on. Faced with attempts by the teachers to modify his behaviour, he was defiantly resistant. He was irresponsive and unreachable" (the speaker went on to say that usually in such cases the cause of the problem was faults in upbringing. Teachers and parents blamed each other...). Michael was thirteen years old, physically underdeveloped and underweight. He still had a whole mouthful of baby teeth and, in addition to this, was not showing any signs of puberty.

We had gathered from the literature that, with the onset of puberty, behavioural difficulties would largely disappear. We had been able to observe this in another child with behaviour problems. We hoped to bridge the time until the onset of puberty with persuasion, remedial teaching and, if necessary, by repeating another year of school.

At the beginning of 1975, while I was going through some old papers, I came across an article about the 'Feingold diet'. Californian allergist Ben F Feingold had ascertained that the particular allergen-free food in the Allergy Clinic of the Kaiser Research Foundation in San Francisco had resulted in a noticeable and distinct improvement in children with difficult behaviour. At that time it was not possible for us to find out the exact kinds of food involved. In July 1975 we obtained Feingold's book 'Why your Child is Hyperactive', published in New York in 1974. Feingold referred among other things to the close connection between carbonated drinks (soft drinks) and behaviour difficulties. We discovered that phosphate was added to these drinks (phosphoric acid gives them a fresher taste). In 1953 Lauersen had irresponsibly announced, after testing only two people, that such additives were harmless.

We wanted to act on Feingold's advice immediately and tried as much neutral baby and toddler food as possible, for example infant milk, baby rusks and bottled toddler food. After the first week it was already evident that this food had a positive effect on our boy but in the long run it would not be possible to feed an almost fourteen year old exclusively on baby food. I thought things over; if colour and flavouring substances were considered to be noxious, they would have to be found among the permitted colourings and flavourings in Germany. There are far fewer of them in Germany than in the USA.

In 1973 'Newsweek' reported a connection between hot dogs and behaviour difficulties. So if 'hot dogs' could trigger behaviour difficulties, then the trigger factors we were looking for had to be found in them. In this context only phosphate came to mind because it is used as a mineral salt in the production of sausages.

For one week we gave our son specially prepared meat without the phosphate additive. He quietened down and was very much improved during that time. Although it tasted rather dry, Michael ate the meat with pleasure, particularly after the insipid baby food. At the end of this week we gave him 250g of an ordinary sausage, half of it on Saturday, the other half on Sunday. On Saturday, about two hours after lunch, Michael started to become restless and to wander aimlessly around the house. He did not know what to do with himself. In the evening he lay in bed, unable to sleep. He had gathered around him countless comics, a packet of biscuits and a bottle of lemonade. This was a familiar picture to us. He said miserably: "I cannot sleep." He was visibly unhappy and obviously worried that the old condition would now return. By Sunday afternoon he had again broken several toys. The syndrome had returned.

We immediately put Michael back onto the diet but the condition lasted through Monday and Tuesday. It was not until Wednesday morning that he became 'normal' again. An impressive pattern!

When this happened, our suspicions regarding phosphate became so strong that we now reduced it in all his food. To find out which foods contained phosphate and how much, we exhausted all sources of information. In the summer of 1975 we received a summary of the 1958 legislation, which listed the additive phosphate in foods. Then we learnt of two symposiums, in 1956 and 1957, in which the use of phosphate in food, mainly in meat products, had been discussed.

It is our impression that the use of phosphate increased as butchering techniques changed. If meat is made into sausage immediately, it keeps its tissue fluids during processing and tastes succulent. But when, as it is necessary and customary in large modern abattoirs, the meat is hung for a time before processing, it loses its tissue fluid and the ability to hold added foreign liquids. Adding salts of phosphoric or citric acids is the only way to restore this ability.

In the two symposiums of 1956 and 1957, the only person to express concern about adding phosphate to food was Professor van Genderen from the 'Institute for Volksfoeding' in the Netherlands. Whilst experimenting in his institute with rabbits, he had observed that hardening of the kidneys developed as a consequence of a hyperparathyroidism. Bell et al. confirmed these observations a few years later when they ascertained that calcium was being removed from the bones of animals and humans. However, the chairman of both symposiums, Professor Lang of Mainz, elegantly swept the objections of the Netherlander under the carpet. The use of phosphate as a food additive, especially as a mineral salt in cold-processed meats and sausages, was officially sanctioned by the state. Once again in 1978, even after our observations were published in the first edition of this book, the harmlessness of phosphate additives was once again written into food additive legislation.

From 1975 to 1978 our family life was governed by the volatile moods of our son. We tried to find out which foods contained phosphate as an additive but only in meat products was this reliably declared.

In 1975 we were not aware of the effect of lecithin – we merely looked for bakers' products without the phosphate baking powder and had no misgivings over baking a cake with sixteen eggs. It was our son's relapses which enabled us to identify the harmful foods and thus, step by step, come to an understanding of the situation. We are still learning daily.

When my phosphate book was first published in the autumn of 1978, it not only attracted the attention of affected families but the experts also sat up and took notice. In the scientific, the national and the daily press the public was advised by renowned scholars that phosphate was a vital substance, without which the human organism could not survive. A reduction of phosphate in the diet would, at the very least, produce deficiency symptoms.

The psychiatrist Dr Roy-Feiler was, at the time, very well informed on the subject. In 1977 her circle of patients had drawn her attention to my observations regarding the issue of phosphate. After six months of experimenting with the diet, she requested official permission to test scientifically the children who had been described in my observations. In February 1978 the children underwent double blind tests with the approval of their parents. All those children given food high in phosphate content reacted violently with relapses.

Because it was not possible to standardise the food sufficiently, Roy-Feiler used capsules containing a phosphate buffer solution of pH 6.9 with 75mg PO_4 (an extremely physiological form of phosphate). These were prepared according to Sörensen's directions. The capsules achieved their immediate purpose so precisely that Roy-Feiler could, in the presence of the College of Psychologists, demonstrate relapses after administering phosphate to the children.

The results of the experiment were impressive enough – fifteen children, one of them our son, were tested with phosphate in a double blind study. Two psychiatrists conducted the experiment. Before the test commenced the children had received low-phosphate food at home and had been found to be psychologically unobtrusive. They then exhibited, under the strain of the phosphate, the characteristic symptoms of the brain function disorder, such as hyperactivity, lack of concentration, etc. Our son returned home after the test with an uncontrolled logorrhea (an excessive flow of words). The next morning he was still so disturbed that within two school lessons he had received three hours of detention and several entries in the class discipline book; then, in despair, he had run away. In those days the teachers were still extremely ignorant. Not even a certificate from Dr Roy-Feiler could mitigate school punishments.

In the summer of 1978, the magazine 'Eltern' ('Parents') interviewed Roy-Feiler. She explained that the children she had tested had displayed a distinct change in their behaviour under the influence of phosphate, although as yet only a limited number of children had undergone the tests. This work was to be continued and the results published at the end of 1978.

On 11 December 1978 Roy-Feiler made her results known at a conference that was held at the German Ministry of Health in Berlin. I, as the person responsible for the discovery, was specifically excluded. Each participant at the conference received a copy of Roy-Feiler's thesis. The recommendations made at that conference were

not considered acceptable then and, even today, they are barred
from publication.

After this incident Roy-Feiler's funding was decreased and her
colleagues persuaded to leave. At the beginning of May 1979, the
newly appointed director prohibited her from doing any work that
dealt with the phosphate problem. She had to turn away all patients
who had made an appointment with her. She was not permitted to
order any more low-phosphate food from the clinic kitchen and was
even prohibited to talk to me. Then her ward was closed and she had
to take over a new position elsewhere.

Today neither Prof Rottka from the BGA (German Federal
Ministry of Health) nor her immediate superior, Prof Glatzel, are
prepared to admit that these events even occurred. It had been
decided at the Berlin conference to investigate my discoveries of the
effects of phosphate. This investigation was conducted by Prof
Spranger and his colleagues Dr Walther and Dr Dieterich in the
Children's Hospital of the University of Mainz. They did not describe
the meals and food given to the subjects and the tests were conducted in such a way that it was inevitable that they would contradict our
experiences.

Nevertheless, to the detriment of those affected, these results
were sufficient for the German Federal Ministry of Health to reject
all approaches concerning the issue of phosphate-sensitivity for the
next ten years.

I voiced my objections to the methods of Prof Spranger and
his colleagues in the 'Deutsche Monatsschrift für Kinderheilkunde'
('German Monthly Magazine for Child Medicine', 1981, p. 56/57).
It is an absolute requirement for the successful outcome of a test
that the ADD-children first must be rendered free of symptoms
through a low-phosphate diet. Otherwise an additional dose of
phosphate in the presence of an already existing syndrome produces
no further symptoms and no valid results can be obtained.

The tests in the Mainz Children's Hospital used an elimination diet that did not correspond with the requirements, i.e. it is a prerequisite that trigger doses of phosphate must be eliminated before testing. At the same time the patient's diet must not be a 'starvation-diet'. Furthermore, the tests did not take into consideration the fact that each reaction lasts for three days.

Last but not least, it needs to be emphasised that being treated in a hospital is stressful for a patient. This can change a subject's reactions to the point where all symptoms of phosphate-sensitivity disappear. The results reported by Adler, Los Angeles, need to be pointed out in this context. At a congress of the John F Kennedy Clinic, John Hopkins University, 1981, Baltimore, Adler informed me that he had made the same observations as I. We had both traced the problem back to adrenergic receptors (up to that point in time Adler had treated more than 30,000 ADD-children).

The research team led by Spranger published their results in the 'Deutsche Monatsschrift für Kinderheilkunde' in 1980, p 382. In my opinion this investigation was flawed and poorly conducted. Unfortunately it was conducted under the auspices of the German Federal Ministry of Health, which has made it more difficult to make progress on the issue.

In the autumn of 1980 in a Bavarian television program, the paediatrician Dr Flade and the psychologist Christoph-Lemke discussed the ADD-syndrome, its causes and effects and also the relevance of low-phosphate food. The radio station received almost two thousand inquiries following the discussion – convincing evidence of the large number of people concerned and their vital interest in the subject.

In the television discussion Dr Flade pleaded for the diet as a result of his experience, whilst Christoph-Lemke advocated the use of psychotherapy. Both are desirable for the diet has a somatic effect and psychotherapy helps the ADD-children to cope more successfully with their disorder. The Swiss specialist in the field of preventative medicine, Dr Vuille of Berne, also commented on the value of psychotherapy when he was interviewed in 1983 on Swiss television.

Over the last few years I too have had many opportunities to present my experiences to interested audiences – to the Social Division of the MIGROS in Lugarno, Adult Education Classes in Sindelfingen, the Consumer Co-operative in Carlsruhe and at the annual meeting of Swiss teachers and speech therapists for children with special needs.

In the period that followed, new cases in various communities were described to me, which confirmed the observations we had already made or revealed interesting new ones. We had earlier discussed how phosphate causes a metabolic alkalosis in a phosphate-sensitive person, which also becomes detectable in the blood and saliva. The mother of two phosphate-sensitive children therefore measured the pH-value of their saliva. It became very obvious to her that a massive shift towards alkalosis set in after her children had eaten nuts. The normal values lie between pH 6.0 and 7.0. The children's values shifted up to pH 9.0, which is a value that to my knowledge has not as yet been described in the literature. Not even carefully devised tests aimed at influencing the saliva had been observed to cause such extreme shifts.

The monitoring of the pH-value of the saliva has proved its worth. Simple distilled cider, wine or even plain white vinegar can remedy an alkalosis if a teaspoon to a tablespoon of vinegar, diluted with water, is administered once or several times a day. In recent times it has been confirmed that vinegar, just as Fazekas has reported of simple mineral salts (1935 – 1974), can influence the hormonal metabolism over and beyond the period of its application. Vinegar stabilises the acid-base balance. As vinegar has been used as a food for thousands of years, we have no misgivings about reporting these experiences. It has also been established that it makes sense to give vinegar in the evening – people have reported falling off to sleep more easily and having a more relaxed night's sleep.

Care must be taken with sport and other forms of physical activity! Phosphate-sensitive children gain their energy more or less exclusively through oxidation. They breathe out so much carbon dioxide that they develop an alkalosis, which is sufficient to cause a relapse. These children are endangered by all influences that affect their acid-base balance as a result of too much oxygen (e.g. hyper-ventilation). Relapses are also brought about by significant changes: for example moving to a new locality, climatic variations, after the resolution of a stressful situation or after taking antibiotics. Vinegar, diluted with water, rectifies the problem and is extremely useful as a simple solution.

In 1981 a father drew my attention to an advertisement for aluminium hydroxide tablets which are used to lower the phosphate blood level. There are two trade names: Aludrox and Antiphosphate. It is possible to substitute these for Ritalin. However, the diet must not be replaced by the taking of tablets. Normal diets never have 'too little' phosphate, but these tablets can remove arbitrary amounts of phosphate from the system, which might result in a phosphate deficiency.

In actual fact the tablets are an indication that the behaviour disorder of ADD-children is caused by an excess of phosphate.

It can also be gathered from the reports received that adult members of families – for example rigid, stubborn and domineering fathers and grandfathers or discontented, quarrelsome mothers – have changed totally under the effect of the diet. They became friendlier, more loving, more cheerful, more sympathetic and no longer came across as intolerant and aggressive.

Recent observations have indicated that cow's milk can trigger ADD in infants. As cow's milk contains six times as much phosphate as human milk, the combination of one third cow's milk and two thirds infant formula still contains too much cow's milk. This is the food mothers habitually gave their infants to supplement their breast milk.

Cow's milk is adjusted to the requirements of a calf that gains a hundred pounds in the same time that a human infant gains fifteen.

People generally assume that the ratio of calcium to phosphate is optimal in milk but the metabolism of calcium is controlled by phosphate. If the human organism is supplied with too much phosphate, the parathyroid hormone is stimulated with the result that calcium is removed from bone matter, irrespective of the level of calcium contained in the food.

The concept that it is solely the ratio of Ca:P[5] which is decisive appears to be a naïve arithmetical assumption. It does not take into consideration all the complicated regulatory mechanisms, which operate independently for calcium and for phosphate. Thus one capsule of frubiase calcium, which contains 47mg phosphoric acid alongside 500mg calcium gluconate and 350mg calcium lactate (except vitamin D) will inevitably trigger a relapse of ADD, despite the fact that the amount of calcium far outweighs that of phosphate.

Phosphate is often added to hard water to soften it. This water is used in infant food. The water supply authorities add 5mg phosphate per litre of water, which is not harmful because of careful supervision. On the other hand, however, private installations in isolated residential premises can accumulate dangerous amounts of phosphate.

Behavioural problems, which are frequently and increasingly evident in infants and toddlers after hospital treatment, are not due to lack of mother love but are the consequence of antibiotic treatment. Antibiotics disrupt the acid-base balance. Just like phosphate, they produce an alkalosis. Lactic acid and vinegar can rectify the

---

6: *1 gram P (phosphorus) is equivalent to approximately 3 grams*
   PO_4 (phosphate)

disrupted balance but not citric acid, nor the presence of the mother in the room.

Even today, as the Kurpfalz-investigation by the Central Institute for Mental Health ascertained, it is a question of developing a conclusive diagnosis of ADD. Neither that Institute nor the Children's Hospital in Mainz could confirm or provide an objective description of the syndrome, although it has been described worldwide in the same way as we have described it.

Doctor Silvia Franz reported: "My patient W K has been under my supervision since 1986, at first only via his mother, his lawyer and by correspondence. At the age of sixteen he committed a robbery and then, while on parole, he committed a second serious larceny which involved deprivation of a victim's liberty. During this period he lived predominantly on coke and hamburgers. He drove around in a stolen car for several days and was soon arrested. He was sentenced to four years' detention, the longest sentence which can be given to juveniles.

"Most of this sentence he had to serve, despite all our endeavours to have his sentence reduced by having his phosphate-sensitivity and food allergies taken into consideration. No doctor from the Phosphate-League was summonsed by the court to give an opinion. Only after I made representations to the Wiesbaden Ministry of the Interior was it possible to arrange for him to at least receive some of his prescribed medication from the prison doctor – but the dose was too low. It is extremely difficult to arrange special diets for prisoners. He, however, very soon noticed which foods were not good for him. He lost a lot of weight because he no longer wanted to eat the foods that caused his severe irritability.

"The Mannheim 'Institute for Mental Illness' could not find any extenuating circumstances to justify a reduced sentence. Surprisingly, a few weeks ago he was released from prison; he now only eats the food that is good and healthy for him and he has already gained six kilograms."

With the orthodox medical establishment refusing to recognise and acknowledge phosphate-sensitivity and its consequences, only very limited help can be expected for such individuals – meaning that it can only come from the next of kin.

The chemical reduction of phosphate with aluminium hydroxide and the control of the acid-base balance now offer possibilities for testing which we could only dream of in the past. They yield concrete numerical data, which can be obtained from the symptom free and healthy child and compared with data from the child suffering from phosphate intoxication, i.e. by conventional clinical comparative methods.

Since 1980 support groups, which counsel and aid afflicted parents when they start introducing the low-phosphate diet, have formed in Germany and Switzerland. These groups want to do neither research work nor therapy. When the families have learned how to adopt the diet, they go back to living the lives of normal private citizens. The more unobtrusively they can live their lives the happier they are.

However, in the meantime a great deal of valuable information has been obtained from these support groups, so that now the damage caused by phosphate can be described precisely.

Many teachers have contributed to these observations. These extremely difficult and quite often not very lovable children, who are incapable of learning, are sitting in their classrooms. They appear to use their undoubted intelligence only to make themselves unpopular. When the diet changes the teachers witness the 'miracle' – little devils suddenly metamorphose into friendly, lovable children. One is reminded of old stories of the changeling and the transformation of personalities in which the same theme is found.

The phosphate problem was revealed and the momentum maintained by private initiatives. Some impression was even made on the hospitals where most of the severely affected children are found.

Government mental hospitals are handicapped by low budgets and inadequate resources and generally are, as a result, reduced to institutions in which people are only locked away without any serious attempt at treatment.

The State Hospital in Marl reported on twenty-two children who participated in a test of the low-phosphate diet. One of these children, who was brain-damaged, did not respond to the change of diet. The other children ceased to be aggressive and regained the ability to communicate verbally.

When the children were given a normal breakfast on the twenty-ninth day, the familiar problems returned within half an hour

It would have been possible to normalise all these children by diet alone. It was unnecessary to hospitalise them, as long as the parental home was willing and able to provide the child with a low-phosphate diet. Unfortunately, this is where the problem lies. Parents are not always willing and able to provide the right conditions. In this context the Government is urged to take a stand on the subject of phosphate.

On 16 January 1988, at the annual meeting of the Swiss Phosphate-League, Dr Andreas Schneider, a paediatrician in Basle, reported on his experiences with the diet. In the Canton Hospital in Winterthür he had conducted a strictly controlled series of tests under scientific conditions. He had observed how the behaviour of his in-patients became normal after eating low-phosphate food and also that the change in behaviour was linked to the pH-value of the saliva. The pH level dropped as their behaviour improved from a relatively alkaline value (approximately one pH unit) to the acid region. Dr Schneider also observed that drug addicts are generally believed to have behaviour problems before they begin to take drugs. This confirms our suspicion that drug addiction is a form of escape from depression and behaviour disorders.

Ritalin creates an acidosis in the same way as the opium

derivatives do; this immediately puts a stop to the discontent and restlessness of the individual whose behaviour is severely disturbed (and brings on dental caries!)[7]. On the basis of our experience we are of the opinion that the regrettably high failure rate in detoxification programs for drug addicts is to be explained by the fact that the patient experiences again the old sense of low self-esteem, which led him to turn to drugs in the first place. Therefore, withdrawal treatment can only be successful if the patient can obtain a sense of well-being by means of a low-phosphate diet.

Dr Schneider mentioned in his report that during examinations close attention was paid to the careful assessment of brain function. The results lay within normal ranges. There were also no records of incidents in the perinatal period, meaning that the children had had no birth defects. The results of computer-tomograms were unexceptional. Schneider believed that heredity most probably caused the behaviour disorder.

We agree with this assessment. The susceptibility to phosphate-sensitivity is inherited and handed down with the type of metabolism.

A few years ago a group connected with Spranger and Steinhausen conceived of a link between paternal alcoholism and the disorders which afflicted the children of alcoholic parents. Because of this, these children were relegated to the category of defective and insignificant individuals. However, we have interpreted this relationship the other way round. The fathers took refuge from their feelings of discontent in alcoholism. Alcoholism is the result of the paternal generation's phosphate-intoxication and is not the cause of brain damage and behaviour problems in their offspring. Here cause and effect were transposed.

7: *Today dental caries has largely ceased to be a problem due to extensive preventative fluoride treatment.*

1.2 CASES WHICH CONFIRM THIS DISCOVERY – BIOGRAPHIES OF ADD-CHILDREN

PARENTS REPORT SUCCESS IN USING THE DIET.
(The following reports were taken from letters and telephone calls to the author)

NORBERT
A pale, difficult eight-year-old boy, who took frubiase calcium capsules prescribed by his doctor. He became extraordinarily restless, fidgeted, could not concentrate – was even less responsive than before the course of treatment. The exacerbation of his symptoms ceased after he stopped taking the medication. Norbert behaved completely normally after being put on the low-phosphate diet.

FRIEDRICH
A ten year old with ADD symptomatology. Medical diagnosis – minimal early childhood brain damage, EEG normal. Attracted attention from the age of three onwards as a result of coordination problems. Increased motor restlessness was followed by psychological disorders. In 1977 his condition improved considerably. There were relapses after changes to his diet. His mother recognised the connection between eating certain foods and the relapses. These foods were the same as the 'forbidden' foods of the low-phosphate diet. From 1978 onwards Friedrich received the low-phosphate diet. Four years later his mother reported, "The problems are all gone – my son is doing well".

ARTHUR
When Arthur was two years old the comment "Severe behaviour disorders" was recorded in his Child Heath Record. After a normal babyhood he became unstable and aggressive. Sedatives caused him to be restless at night; he was even more fidgety during the day. He

pulled flowers to pieces, threw eggs which he had taken from the fridge, tormented pets, bit himself and others – was incapable of being gentle. The neighbours complained. The paediatrician referred the parents to a psychotherapist. Many hours of therapy brought no improvement. Inspired by an article in 'Stern' (No. 40, 21.9.1978), the parents changed the boy's diet to bottled baby food. They gave him no sweets or chocolate. After one day only he began to improve.

Later we heard that Arthur had turned eight years old. By that time he was living with his grandmother as his parents had divorced. His mother also had had behaviour problems during her childhood and adolescence. He was kept on a restricted diet. Yoghurt and ice-cream caused relapses.

SVEN

Because of his behaviour disorders it had been proposed to transfer Sven to a school for problem children. With the introduction of a low-phosphate diet and the assistance of an understanding teacher this course of action became unnecessary. Whenever he suffered a relapse the teacher sent Sven home immediately, so that the cause could be determined.

In 1979 he left primary school and attended a junior high school. Here, Sven suffered severe relapses after buying soft drinks from a vending machine. There have been no problems with Sven's behaviour since these drinks have been eliminated from his diet.

MARKUS

Had seen doctor after doctor from the age of two – all in vain. Ritalin and the Wiedemann-treatment brought no relief. In October 1978, by which time Markus was nineteen, his mother read the article published in 'Stern' about phosphate-sensitive children. She encouraged her son to try the diet. The diet was effective. Markus felt well. He and his family were worried about a relapse occurring during the time that he had to serve in the German Federal Armed Forces (compulsory in Germany). It would be difficult for him to stick to the diet in the army.

MARTIN

'Grunted like a pig' through his nose. Sinusitis was treated with penicillin. Although the inflammation subsided, his overall condition deteriorated. Bilateral otitis media (middle ear inflammation) was treated with penicillin. Medical treatment continued because of discharge from the eustachian tubes. The doctor considered the grunting a 'silly habit', especially as Martin frequently displayed 'ticks' (he blinked his eyes, spat, pulled up his shirt, all his muscles were in constant movement).

He did well at school but his behaviour was strange. The psychiatrist found nothing wrong with him; his EEG was normal. Martin was given relaxation therapy and sedatives – without success. Even a course of forty Ritalin tablets brought no change. He woke several times a night, ran around the house crying and screaming. It was not possible to communicate with him during the nightly episodes and he had no recollection of anything the next day. "It was as if his body was electrified".

Then the doctor diagnosed Attention Deficit Disorder. Martin was treated with A-Mulsin, Ergenyl and homeopathic remedies. The parents sought advice because of difficulties caused by his insolent, aggressive behaviour at school.

At this point, a doctor referred the mother to me. She was given the phosphate book. In October 1982 during a meeting of the Phosphate-League, Martin's mother reported that the boy was doing well. The 'ticks' and the 'grunting' had disappeared. He was continuing to stick to the diet.

MATTHIAS

This eleven-year-old was restless and acted in a strange way. He
became irritable whenever he was in a group. He needed to be alone,
required peace and quiet, and space to run. He suffered from
circulatory problems, hypotension, heart rhythm and sleep disorders,
had motor restlessness, was aggressive, called his mother an "old
witch" and screamed, "I hate you!" He changed totally after a week
on the diet. The diet was supplemented with a small dose of Ritalin
during school. In 1981 he received an outstanding school report
from the junior high school. This family also noticed that the father
had changed as a result of the diet. A rather cold and uncompro-
mising man had become friendly and sympathetic and the troubled
marriage was saved.

EGON

In 1976 the family moved into a house with a phosphate filter to
soften the water. Egon was born in August 1976. He developed
indigestion, heartburn, sleep disorders and – after consuming cocoa,
chocolate, oats and raisins – diarrhoea. At the age of one his
adenoids were removed and his condition improved slightly. At the
end of June 1978, the chemical reservoir of the water-softening
device was empty and the filter was filled with tap water. The boy's
digestion normalised.

During 1979 Egon suffered from diarrhoea again and from
pains in the legs; he could hardly walk. The paediatrician could not
detect any anomalies. Diarrhoea also occurred after he ate whole-
grain bread and ice-cream; he could not tolerate stewed fruit,
peaches or carrots. Egon had phases of aggression. He was
hyperactive, stuttered and was provocative during gymnastics lessons.
He had taken to wetting and soiling himself again. When his mother
heard of the low-phosphate diet and started using it, Egon's
condition improved. Relapses occurred only when he ate the wrong

things. From 1980 onwards the diet was followed strictly and from that time on Egon continued to feel well.

OTTWIN

Attracted attention in primary school-exercise books were missing or torn, rubbers and pencils destroyed and pen-nibs splayed. Ottwin displayed aggressive behaviour and 'clowned around' during lessons. Baby food improved his behaviour-relapses occurred with a normal diet. He attended a secondary boarding school, which did not improve his behaviour. Ottwin had to be fetched home again.

In 1978 Ottwin received three months of clinical psychiatric treatment. The clinic refused a request that he be given a low-phosphate diet. Ottwin displayed a lot of anxiety after this treatment. Then the mother started to give the boy the low-phosphate diet. This brought the first signs of success. The local secondary school reported "working cooperatively" and "exemplary behaviour".
A change back to the senior high school meant that Ottwin had to travel a long way to school, which tempted him to eat sweets and drink coke. Whenever he drank coke, he suffered severe relapses; each one lasted for three days. As a supplement to the diet, Ottwin was prescribed Ritalin. The effects of the medication were unpredictable. Ottwin tired easily and did not pay proper attention in class. Occasionally his behaviour at school was atrocious, whereas at home there was no reason for complaint. A further test indicated that Ottwin was highly phosphate-sensitive and needed to stay on the strictest diet.

HEINZ

An adopted child, four years old, very pale with sensitive skin, weak muscles, flatulence, testicles not descended – otherwise healthy. He craved attention and affection. He broke toys. His hands were never still and he chattered incessantly. Heinz could not leave adults in peace, demanding their constant attention. He also behaved in group situations in such a way that he needed supervision. He failed to relate with other children and the kindergarten refused to enrol him.

Heinz was manually clumsy and had problems coordinating his limbs. He had trouble standing and running. He often fell over and had little staying power. He ate excessively, especially meat and sweets but no vegetables. Heinz could think logically. He could talk his way out of anything; when he did not like something, he always managed to avoid it. He had little interest in learning, poor ability to concentrate and could not retain anything. His speech development was retarded. He had problems with articulation (speech muscles) as well as difficulties with word choices and grammar.

After the introduction of the low-phosphate diet, Heinz was able to play on his own for a long period of time. He drew his first pictures, no longer antagonised people, was calmer and more at peace with himself, went to bed more quietly without screaming and no longer presented a problem. When the diet was interrupted (so that the kindergarten teacher could be convinced that it was a vital necessity) a relapse occurred. The teacher requested that the diet be continued, otherwise she "couldn't put up with it (i.e. the boy's behaviour after eating normal food!) any more!"

HERBERT

This sixteen-year-old "kept strictly to the diet" after reading the 'Stern'. His whole personality changed for the better. His ability to concentrate improved, he related much better to other family members and his motivation and ability to stay on task increased significantly. 'Lapses' were unavoidable (the hurdle was chocolate...). Recently Herbert had taken up horse-riding; he handled the horse brilliantly but said, "I can't handle the horse when I've been nibbling". After experiencing difficulties at grammar school, he changed to a comprehensive secondary school and subsequently enjoyed going to school.

BERND

Before Bernd tried the diet, he was academically about two years
behind at school. His participation in class improved markedly after
going on the low-phosphate diet – Bernd was able to copy writing
from the blackboard, making only a few mistakes (even in English!).
He also took part in after school activities. He had relapses after
eating sauerkraut and a big helping of scrambled egg. "Everything
was as before. He could not copy down words any more; his writing
was barely legible. He no longer made eye contact; his laughter
disappeared. Instead he was quick to cry and complain the moment
any demands were made on him. He kept to himself, slept poorly
and started bed-wetting again. Thus the relapse made it very clear
how essential the diet was and that it was the only thing that brought
about... a positive change".

SUSANNE

Went onto the diet in 1981. Her aggression and inattentiveness
lessened considerably after only a fortnight. Milk caused a relapse.
She stopped drinking milk (two and a half cups a day) and taking
Dienaplex drops which was prescribed by a doctor and once again
became happy and contented. Her parents reported: "For us this all
seems like a miracle... at last we can breathe a sigh of relief. This very
sensitive child is doing well, as long as she keeps to the diet."

KLAUS

He was thirteen years old and had only been on the diet for a few
weeks. For the first time in his life he was able to say something
positive about himself: "I always woke up in such a bad mood, which
lasted all day long" and "I want to go on feeling good like this!"
Klaus could now chat with friends, listen to music, and was aware
of changes in temperature. He no longer quarrelled with his sister.
In spite of this, the teacher recommended a change to a school for

children with special needs.

His dentist injected the sympathetic hormone epinephrine to reduce the flow of blood. Approximately an hour later a severe relapse occurred, which lasted until the next day. When the next visit to the dentist was due, Klaus was given Ritalin as a prophylactic measure (because it can control the epinephrine reaction). After five hours it was necessary to give Klaus another dose of 5mg of Ritalin and again the following morning.

DETLEF

He was a problem child from a dysfunctional family. Detlef's sister – a medical practitioner – read the article in 'Stern' about the ADD-children. The symptoms of the children described were the same as those of her brother. He too was hyperactive, with low physical endurance, was unable to concentrate and suffered from generalised anxiety.

Detlef passed the school entrance test extremely well and started school normally. His first reports were good. Then he changed. Problems with teachers and fellow students increased and his level of achievement went down. Two psychologists were consulted – without success. From grade four onwards in primary school, Detlef was assessed as having behaviour problems. Despite this, he was accepted into the junior high school. Further problems developed – he had to sit alone, his level of achievement dropped. First trial with the diet – he responded. A relapse occurred when he ate a non-permitted Wiener sausage, which taught Detlef that he had no choice but to follow the diet faithfully. Other foods that are 'permissible in small quantities' were eliminated after he experienced sporadic relapses.

With the aid of the diet Detlef's level of achievement stabilised in the first year; it even started to improve. Three years after being introduced to the diet he was managing to stay in the top half of his class. A restless but lethargic, indifferent boy was transformed into an exceptionally active child, well liked by teachers and fellow students alike. The letter read: "What thrills us most is that the atmosphere in the family has also improved. Detlef's wit and cheerfulness are highly contagious. Our problem child has changed into a wonderful human being who brightens up our days. It is impossible to describe how happy we are because of the changes created by reading the information in your book."

ALFRED

Was a well-balanced, quiet child until he turned two. Then he was admitted to hospital for laryngitis; he developed pneumonia and was prescribed antibiotics. An anxious, tearful child arrived home after the hospital stay. Alfred would only go where he could hold his mother's hand – even at night he had to hold her hand. At the age of three and a half he had a tonsillectomy and became a bit more independent (suppurating tonsils cause permanent stress!).

Alfred attracted attention in the kindergarten. He had no knowledge of colours, numbers or letters when he started school. He was obviously retarded compared with his younger sister. Despite learning difficulties at primary school – he took a long time to do his homework – his performance placed him in the top third of his class. Alfred was anxious, helpless, pedantic, lacked the ability to make decisions and to concentrate, showed little consideration for others and was subject to mood swings. At the age of seven he began to stutter. He managed to be accepted into the grammar school but he needed more and more time to complete his homework.

In 1977 he started on the diet (which was then at a rather rudimentary stage). His stuttering decreased and after a time it completely disappeared. His ability to concentrate, memorise and comprehend improved considerably. Alfred went to the top of the class. Occasional relapses made it crystal clear to Alfred how phosphate in food affected him. Abruptly he would become unmanageable, talk in a subdued way or whine, and become impervious to reason. The last relapse occurred in the summer of 1982 after drinking just a single cup of cocoa (after four years free of problems).

INGE

Twelve years old, an only child. A congenital hip problem was treated successfully. Her motor development was delayed as a toddler; at the age of eighteen months she could neither walk nor talk. The Tübingen University Clinic diagnosed her as a 'late developer'. At the age of twenty months Inge started to walk but often fell over; she was noticeably restless and fidgety. The Psychiatric Clinic for Children diagnosed brain damage and predicted that she would have to attend a special school – she was prescribed physiotherapy and speech therapy.

When she was five, Inge was still using sign language to make herself understood. She attended kindergarten for four years and was given speech therapy. At the age of eight and a half she enrolled in a school which had a standard curriculum and offered speech therapy. In grade two there were complaints about inattentiveness, fidgetiness and restlessness. Inge was incapable of working independently, did not do her homework and disrupted the class. The family doctor prescribed Pyrithioxine (Encephabol) to calm her – it had the opposite effect. The medication was stopped. Occasionally she became absent minded. The Psychiatric Clinic for Children detected in the EEG a strong tendency to seizures. The results from the computer tomogram provided no information. Daily doses of Ergenyl prevented seizures. Inge repeated grade three without success. It was thought likely that she would have to attend a special school.

When Inge tried the diet, she became calmer, more balanced and coherent. The child could now play by herself, was cooperative, sang to herself, drew bright, cheerful pictures. Relapses occurred after eating two pieces of bread with Lyon's sausage and cheese cake (baked with six eggs). Transfer to a school for children with learning disabilities became unavoidable. Generally she had become, as the teacher also confirmed, much calmer and more balanced.

KURT

Eighteen years old, he had been expelled from several schools, including a boarding school. He was considered "unfit for a boarding school". An apprenticeship was also problematical. An experiment with aluminium hydroxide tablets normalised his behaviour. He went back to boarding school. Kurt became polite and friendly. He passed his driving test. Kurt had to rely on aluminium hydroxide tablets because it was not possible for him to keep to a low-phosphate diet in boarding school.

JÖRG

Twenty years old; suffered from behaviour disorders, dyslexia and speech problems. Every time he tried to speak, he shouted loudly (he could suppress the shouting for a short time when it became exceptionally embarrassing for him!). The compulsion to shout disappeared with the diet. Relapses occurred after consuming ice-cream and cocoa. Jörg was given aluminium hydroxide tablets to eliminate the remaining symptoms of ADD (the inclination to play the clown for others).

HERMANN AND HANNA

Adopted children, born in wedlock, neglected. They were three and four years old respectively at the time of their adoption. Neither child could speak – they communicated with each other in a kind of baby talk. When Hermann was five he started talking incessantly, raging and screaming, even at kindergarten. When punished he would howl in his bedroom. At night he would sit in bed crying; in the morning he would wake up sobbing. Sedatives hyped him up even more. He was pale of complexion and remained thin despite the good food he ate. When he was ill and scarcely ate, Hermann amazed his parents by behaving normally. In 1979 they tried the low-phosphate diet for three months but Hermann did not respond.

Hanna developed into a tall, quiet girl. She only gradually recovered from her speech deficiency. She was very afraid of being touched, went rigid and clenched her jaw if anyone tried to pick her up.

Both children's teeth were totally free of caries. In 1981 the diet was reintroduced; for Hanna it was an absolute success. She became friendly and sociable; she was able to attend a comprehensive secondary school. Hermann too ceased to cause problems at school, he became considerate towards his sister and displayed completely normal behaviour. Relapses occurred when they ate the wrong things.

SPECIAL LETTERS AND REPORTS:

1. On 11 March 1980, the mother of an afflicted child wrote to the Federal Executive for Economic Information in Bonn. As a result of the 'Stern' report, she had bought the phosphate book and tested the recommended diet on her son. She had an especially good opportunity to do this, as she was able to buy exactly the right foods in an American PX-shop. Here is a quotation from her letter: "The remarkable and striking success of the diet was so amazing that I could hardly believe it was the same child. The success was obvious within the first month and was apparent to his teacher too."
    The writer requested the Executive to use all its influence to make it compulsory for food manufacturers to label every ingredient in food. It was difficult to keep to the diet without such a system of

labelling. Moreover, it was of paramount importance to drastically reduce the amount of phosphate additives. The letter writer commented on the significance and necessity of the diet for ADD-children, in particular when they experienced a relapse. She said 'torture' would be the right word to describe what these children had to endure.

2. On 14 January 1980, a woman from Hanau, who had – on her own initiative – introduced mothers of children with behavioural difficulties to our diet, wrote to the Children's Diet Research Institute in Dortmund and reported the following: Mothers, who had kept their children on the diet for several weeks, had observed a "striking improvement in their behaviour which was evident to everyone". But "the improvement was frequently interrupted by relapses lasting several days that were occasioned by consuming certain foods." She went on to say: "According to our observations it appears that the syndrome is at its worst when a certain phosphate level is exceeded. The children are then barely responsive, hyperactive, uncaring, inattentive, have difficulties in falling asleep and so on."

3. Report by a psychologist dated 17 October 1981: An eleven-year-old boy had severe behaviour disorders with compulsive restlessness. He displayed impulsive, indiscriminate aggression, which he directed against his school and the parental home. The EEG disclosed cerebral hyperactivity (there had been birth complications). An intelligence test revealed ability well below the average, close to mental retardation. His concerned and conscientious parents put him on the diet, which they followed very precisely; a few days later they perceived an enormous improvement in their son's behaviour. A week later the boy helped himself to chips and coke at a cornershop when he was

hungry. That very evening all the behaviour disorders resurfaced, including difficulty in going to sleep. After this incident, the boy kept to the diet and about six months later he appeared to be almost normal. His behaviour and performance at school had improved considerably too.

4. Excerpt from a report by paediatrician Dr Ursula Klemm on the subject: 'Attention Deficit Disorder in Children' in 'Der Kinderarzt' ('The Paediatrician') of December 1983:

"... I have employed, despite being very dubious about it, Hertha Hafer's low-phosphate therapy, although I am aware of the various papers, which attempt to demonstrate – by referring to chemical and statistical analyses – that this therapy cannot be effective!

"On the contrary, I have discovered that the experiments I have made with the diet in my practice have been very – and sometimes unbelievably – successful. I have also observed relapses that were caused by eating the wrong foods. But why one glass of coke or one slice of a cake baked with baking powder, containing a relatively small quantity of phosphate, can trigger such a remarkable relapse I can no more explain than can the various institutes of food chemistry. To be convinced one only has to have experienced it.

"I am only too well aware that mainstream medicine disapproves of this therapy but, to help these children and their families, I would like to encourage doctors to let their patients try it, particularly as the diet is totally harmless and is not deficient in vitamins. The resultant successes will justify this step even though in the present state of our knowledge there is no scientific explanation for why the diet works.

"... My experience involving many cases confirms that a

hyperactive, severely behaviour-disturbed child can demonstrate dramatic changes with enormous improvement in behaviour after three to four days on the diet. He or she can suddenly listen, concentrate, be considerate, be coherent and be in a good mood. But it can take ten to fourteen days before some children respond positively.

"When the wrong kind of food is eaten, however, the previous – often intolerable – condition recurs after twenty to sixty minutes, which happens as surely as if it were a law of nature! More than anything else, I consider the relapses after eating the wrong food to be the absolute proof of Hertha Hafer's method."

Fortunately, in the mean time, some institutions have begun to provide their students with low-phosphate food when requested.

The boarding school at Fredeburg, W. Kling, Kapellenstrasse 5-8, D-57392 Schmallenberg-Fredeburg is a conventional institution which caters for children who require low-phosphate food.

The Ev. Kinderheim in Celle is a home for children suffering from emotional stress. They report very good results with the low-phosphate food.

The Lehrinstitut Eberhardt in Mainz is an institution that is recommended for juveniles who have overcome their behaviour disorders and who wish to make up for school years they have missed.

Young people who suffer from phosphate-sensitivity are disadvantaged when they live in military accommodation, homes, hospitals or prisons and have to rely on canteens or similar large kitchens for their meals.

2.0 A SCIENTIFIC SURVEY OF THE ADD ISSUE

2.1 DESCRIPTION OF THE SYNDROME: LITERATURE AND OPINION

In the literature worldwide descriptions of the Attention Deficit Disorder syndrome are very consistent. Most of the information comes from the United States of America.

In 1976 Ross and Ross spelt out in their book 'Hyperactivity: Research, Theory and Action' the forms of behaviour that they found in ADD-children. They referred to the following characteristics:

1. Hyperactivity
Incapable of sitting still for more than a few minutes. The children fidget constantly, talk incessantly and 'are into everything'.

2. Lack of Concentration and Distractibility
ADD-children are inattentive, easily distracted, indifferent, careless, act without forethought, have little staying-power and are unable to finish tasks.

3. Social Problems
They relate poorly to others but they nevertheless have much need of reassurance; there are unpredictable displays of affection; they constantly demand attention; they are uncooperative and obstinate. These children cannot play without close adult supervision. They hum, make noises, mutter to themselves and try too hard to please. They cannot handle rejection and disappointment.

4. Fixation of Habits
They adapt with difficulty to changes in their surroundings – have problems integrating into a community and do not comply with

directions, they withdraw from unfamiliar persons and tasks.

5. Aggression
They tease other children and disrupt their activities, are unusually aggressive and are therefore unpopular with peers. They fight; they destroy toys, furniture and other things. The tendency to lie is reported to be a particularly common feature.

Wender, who is considered an expert in behavioural research in the USA, listed in his book 'Minimal Dysfunction in Children', among other things, the following characteristic anomalies in behaviour:

1. High Level of Motor Activity
Wender described a child who displayed restless behaviour in the 'play pen'. He stood up and walked early and then went berserk like a child King-Kong with the result that he almost demolished the parental home. The child 'was into everything', touched and broke all that was accessible to him.
According to Wender's observations older children were constant 'fidgets'. They were themselves aware of the agitation and restlessness and they attributed it to nervousness. Wender also attributed the logorrhea, the continual chatter, to the hyperactivity. Some of the children he described remarked that they couldn't stop thinking even in their sleep.

2. Inattentiveness
Wender claimed that ADD-children do not finish their work properly – they cannot stay on task and are unable to listen – it appears that they do not notice when they are being spoken to. On the other hand, however, they can be obsessive about details. They do not have the ability to discriminate between what is important and what is not. They cling rigidly to their own ideas.

3. Impulsiveness

Destructive behaviour, dishonesty, theft, arson, sexual recklessness, bed-wetting and soiling are the result of an inability to control impulsiveness. Wender also put in this category: the sudden out-pouring of rage when ADD-children do not get their own way; their demands for constant attention; carelessness; chaos and disorgani-sation arising from a lack of forethought; frequent accidents and – last but not least – the anti-social behaviour of juveniles. Wender stated that these children are indiscriminate vandals, compulsive thieves and arsonists. According to him, it is characteristic of these modes of behaviour that they are autonomous and are not subject to the control of that voice of conscience which develops progressively in a normal individual. Consequently these children are often classified as psychopaths. Wender believed that the most important aspect of the entire syndrome is the absence of appropriate control mechanisms.

If one takes into account here MacLean's description of the function of the brain, the conclusion is inescapable that the the unconscious and non-verbal impulses of the older areas of the brain – the brain stem and the limbic system – are not being assessed or controlled by the cerebral cortex.

4. Poor Social Skills

According to Wender ADD-children are unable to form friendships because of their resistance to social expectations, their greater inde-pendence and their extroversion (Eysenck also concurs). Wender considered adjectives such as stubborn, obstinate, negative, bossy, disobedient, unapproachable as typical descriptors of their behaviour and he characterised ADD-children as 'perpetual two year olds'. He knew of no effective corrective measures for their behaviour. Furthermore, according to Wender's observations, their behaviour changes in adolescence from rebelliousness to loneliness with underlying aggression. The ADD-child resists adult control; he or she tries to dominate peers (and for this reason often seeks younger companions). The reason that such children do not have friends is not the result of pathological or schizoid characteristics but is due to their behaviour. Wender further mentioned that it is characteristic of these children that they have no qualms about running away from home. One moment they are craving affection; the next they are aggressively rejecting it.

5. Emotions (Mood Swings)

In the field of emotions, Wender observed important deviations from normal behaviour – ranging from greater instability, irritability, mood swings to a decreased sensitivity to pain. ADD-children do not respond to reproach or punishment, unless it is by avoiding being touched. Babies lie in their cots like 'touch me nots'. Children frequently over-react both in enjoyable and unpleasant situations; they completely lose their self-control, especially in the presence of many people.

Wender also observed that ADD-children react to minor stresses, for example hunger or fatigue, more intensely than other children. According to him any dysphoric sign – a symptom of irritation and uneasiness – is due to their inability to be content. He made another discovery in regard to the obvious anxiety of ADD-children – their anxiety appears to be neurotic and they are often the children of over-organised, rigid parents. They differ from schizoid or brain damaged children who display otherwise similar behavioural anomalies in that their anxiety can be triggered by environmental situations.

Ross and Ross's standpoint is psychiatry, Wender's is paediatrics whereas Carol Whalen and Barbara Hencker, of the South California University in Los Angeles, developed a very thorough classification of symptoms from the perspective of psychology. Rather than listing symptoms, they made a close study of a typical preschool child: The child's mother had not been aware of anything unusual until he turned two. Then there was an outbreak of mumps in his immediate neighbourhood. The sudden development of ADD-symptoms in the child gave reason to believe that he had contracted encephalitis but this suspicion was not confirmed.

The boy was hyperactive and unpredictable. If he was not running, he was jigging up and down or back and forth on his chair. His fine motor skills were impaired; his gross motor movements were clumsy and awkward. If an adult attempted to aid the boy, he was likely to fly at him or her with his fists, raging with fury. If he wished to take a toy off a shelf, he would throw everything else that was on the shelf to the floor. If he saw another child with a toy, he took it off that child.

The child's attention span was, according to Whalen and Hencker, short. He could not listen to the end of stories. Although he had an IQ of 120 (Stanford-Binet), he never seemed to be able to learn from experience. The boy did not cry when he fell, but did so excessively when frustrated with a situation. He would constantly make desperate attempts to get attention. Once he climbed up a tree from which he jumped onto a roof. Then he tried to climb into the chimney and was prevented from doing so only by its narrowness. He was proud that other children had watched this stunt, but the others were unwilling to accept him – they were afraid of him.

The child ran away from the kindergarten several times.

A larger study by Battle and Lacey disclosed that hyperactive boys lack motivation to strive for success. They considered themselves to be unintelligent but were, however, bold, aggressive and possessed of great stamina in physical activities – they gained attention and recognition by means of physical exploits. Psychological tests revealed substantial correlations with the clinical observations.

The research revealed that the attitudes of their mothers to these boys as preschoolers ranged from criticism to rejection. Older children experienced a lack of parental protection. They received serious punishments for disobedience and the mothers were inclined to underestimate their children's intelligence. According to Battle and Lacey, hyperactive girls have it easier – they are less rejected.

Weiss and Hechtmann defined ADD using the following criteria: Relative to age, excessive general hyperactivity or motor restlessness. Impulsive running, climbing and crawling at preschool age and an inability to sit still in primary school; the children jump and fidget. It is difficult for them to pay attention and to complete tasks. They are disorganised in the way they go about projects; they forget requirements or tasks; they behave impulsively and present slipshod work in spite of taking great pains; they talk a lot of nonsense; they disrupt lessons, are unable to wait their turn and they fight with other children because of their low level of tolerance to frustration.

More than other researchers, Weiss and Hechtmann have drawn attention to the fact that problems with people outside the family start at kindergarten age. Acquaintances and friends do not like to have ADD-children in their homes because they touch everything, break things and are constantly disruptive. For this reason they are also not popular with kindergartens.

Weiss and Hechtmann attributed the very obvious problems, which ADD-children experience at school, to educational expectations of the classroom, which they are not capable of meeting. They felt it would be better for someone to take care of such a child in a one-to-one-situation. The most important characteristic of an ADD juvenile is, apart from failure at school, his or her anti-social and immoral behaviour.

A statistical compilation of the results of the survey did not result in an absolutely uniform description of the syndrome – 45.6 per cent were rated as aggressive and 23.4 per cent as hyperactive.

The German researcher Lempp, who sought to describe reasons for failure at school in his book 'Lernerfolg und Schulver-sagen' ('Success and Failure at School'), described nonconformity in the classroom, difficulty in concentrating, a low level of tolerance to frustration and showing off as typical symptoms. He described the children's distractibility and their inattentiveness, but also persever-ance and persistence of attention when it is spontaneous (an ADD-child can be relaxed and absorbed in a book if it is one that is especially interesting to the child, for example, comics which con-tinuously change the subject. If one tries to get the child's attention, he or she immediately starts fidgeting again [Hafer]).

Lempp stated that children raised in children's homes are likely to be hyperactive, whereas children who live with their grandparents tend to be more anxious and compulsive. He concluded that there is a correlation. It is logical to expect that hyperactive children who are troublesome and intolerable will be sent off to children's homes. On the other hand, children with hypoactive behaviour disorders can be expected to be taken care of by grandparents. Thus Lempp reversed cause and effect, but he understood correctly that ADD-children are more likely to be low achievers than normal children. His contention that teachers in particular can have a role in helping these children to achieve greater self-esteem also should be emphasised.

Lempp was the first person to describe in detail one phenom-enon that especially disrupts the routine at school – that of the 'class-clown'. As an ADD-child is unable to secure normal affection, respect or even appreciation within his or her class but craves this very attention and affection, it is highly likely that he or she will employ his or her physical strength or clowning to draw attention to him or herself.

American scientists, who have otherwise made the same observations as we have, have noticed the clown-syndrome much less. Obviously the greater amount of sport which is played in schools in the USA functions as an important relief valve for ADD-children.

It is remarkable that not even paediatricians have much to say about physical characteristics when describing the symptoms of ADD-children. Brower and Mercer, of the Virginia University, however, pointed out that hypoglycaemia exacerbates the ADD-symptoms. They quoted Alabiso, who recognised that the core problem of ADD-children is their inability to pay attention, and Knobel, who characterised the behaviour of these children as 'typically subcortical'. The children demonstrate a poor relationship to reality, they lack control and their physical abilities are impaired. Knobel understood correctly that amphetamines stimulate the cortex's control via subcortical impulses in the brain, i.e. they help control the children's outbursts.

The behavioural therapists Bekker, Engelmann and Thomas (1971) gave their opinion as follows: "The fundamental problem of the hyperactive child is that he or she has not been taught to work consistently at tasks. He or she has not been instructed to persist long enough with a project to be successful. The solution to this problem is to find a way that increases perseverance and the time needed to complete a task". In this publication a number of corrective, therapeutic measures are referred to, for example, removal of the child from the classroom situation into a small group and specific training in perseverance, listening, seeing, thinking before answering. After two days of practice a child displays better results than before.

Cruickshank also advocated this method, which not only ties up enormous amounts of professional time but has not brought and will not bring any lasting results.

Adler (and incidentally Wender as well), who has treated ADD-children with Ritalin (but has also tested the Feingold-diet), characterised the ADD-child as 'in perpetual motion'. He has drawn to our attention the fact that these children squander enormous energy.

He has described an ADD-child as follows: "touches everything and fiddles with every object that is accessible to him, talks in 'outbursts' without thinking, smashes things, attacks other children, can be tense, irritable and aggressive. Emotions vary from tranquillity to panic for no apparent logical reason; there are frequent outbursts of rage; he or she cannot handle rejection. An ADD-child cannot remember anything from one minute to the next. He or she loses his or her possessions and has poor concentration, especially when abstract topics are being discussed. In apparent contrast to the extreme distractibility is his or her compulsive behaviour – he or she continuously repeats the same action over and over."

Normal individuals can assess correctly information that they receive by seeing, hearing and touching. Hyperactive children have 'blind spots' – they cannot evaluate what they see and hear. They are incapable of comprehending the logical structure of a sentence. Although they can describe a picture, they cannot recognise its meaning or copy the simplest outline. Some children lisp or stutter and their hearing is impaired. Poorly developed motor coordination handicaps these children when they try to skip, jump, run in a straight line or catch a ball. They often have difficulty in distinguishing between right and left. Inadequate fine motor skills are often evident when the child is writing. Adler drew the reader's attention to this problem in his book 'Your Overactive Child, How to Help Him'. Adler was motivated to write this book by his awareness of the extraordinarily high number of affected children – 30,000 in twelve years in a single city! According to Adler many ADD-children outgrow their problem – an encouraging prognosis. He queried why then one should be concerned and replied: "Because many of these children are deprived of their opportunities to learn during those crucial years which society has allocated for them to gain the knowledge that they require to master the tasks of life."

A survey of literature would not be complete without mentioning those researchers who attribute ADD to the properties of food. Of these, the best known is Feingold. He described ADD in the same terms as the experts referred to above. And, just like the therapists who work with amphetamines, he observed how the syndrome disappeared as a result of his treatment program. He could therefore, like other researchers, observe and describe a 'normal condition', whereas the psychologists and psychiatrists could only presume a hypothetical 'normal condition'. When a child is treated with Ritalin and the treatment is successful in controlling most of his symptoms, it becomes possible for scientists to define ADD clearly and precisely. They merely have to describe the condition of the child before the therapeutic intervention or that which reappears after the effect of the medication has worn off.

Feingold saw that food influenced the syndrome. He pointed out that he had worked as a paediatrician in clinics and universities over half a lifetime and had not encountered many ADD-cases during that time. In 1945 he became an allergist. Then he noticed that the incidence of ADD was increasing as soft drinks became more widely available in the USA but he firmly rejected allergy as the cause.

In 1972 Feingold began to treat children with a diet that eliminated man-made additives and certain foods. This diet was essentially a low-phosphate diet although it contained a number of foods that, as we have discovered in the meantime, cause relapses, e.g. milk, cocoa, sweet-corn, etc.

One of Feingold's patients was a six-year-old boy (his twelve-year-old brother was not affected) who attracted attention as a baby because he was not affectionate as babies usually are. As a toddler he steered his tricycle straight at cars coming towards him. At school he constantly caused chaos in his class. Clinical examinations provided no hints, no susceptibility to hypoglycaemia, no spasms; only the EEG registered anomalies that pointed to the cerebrum. The boy was neurologically normal. An element of the diagnosis was that the family was experiencing stress. The parents appeared to be firm and principled in their handling of the children. It was suggested that Dilantine (anti-epileptic drug) be tried. Feingold noted that in this case a reduction of the level of stress in the family would be impossible to achieve because such a child would not respond to normal intervention.

Another boy, who was seven years old, had the 'typical' hyperkinetic syndrome with 'soft signs' (an expression for anomalies in performance without somatic manifestations). He was unable to button up his shirt, had poor hand and eye coordination. He was given Ritalin (40mg a day!) and the response was extremely good at first but the boy became sleepy (like a zombie). The response to a lower dose of Ritalin (30 mg) was still good but then one day he again displayed all the ADD-symptoms – restlessness, distractedness, incapacity to adjust to changed circumstances and irritability. The child talked constantly, even when he was supposed to be listening.

A third patient, whom Feingold described, had been receiving Ritalin from the age of three. He was unhappy, extremely hyperactive and uncontrollable. He was unable to keep his mind on one topic for more than three seconds. Ritalin brought relief but, at the age of five – despite Ritalin – problems manifested themselves at school. The boy could not recognise numbers or letters although he was considered 'bright'. He did not get on with his schoolmates and he created chaos in the classroom. Eventually he was prescribed Stelazine (a tranquilliser) in addition to Ritalin. This medication regulated his sleep and improved his muscle control.

The fourth patient, who had a sister in good health, was seventeen years old, tall and well built. He had been hyperactive since early childhood, had smashed his cot and had been a poor sleeper. He behaved like a 'sly fox'. When he was six, his parents observed that he was disorganised. He did not get on with other children. He was unable to achieve success at school, was unable to complete his work and made every effort to attract people's attention to himself. He was treated with Dexedrine (dexamphetamine) at the age of eight. When he turned thirteen he was prescribed Ritalin and Stelazine daily, administered in three doses. The boy's parents and educators had been told that the problem would disappear at puberty. Compared with adolescents of the same age, at seventeen he was developmentally two years behind his peers. The hyperactivity seemed to have lessened but his coordination was as poor as before. The medication had not done any good. The boy was in danger of becoming a complete failure.

Professor Rapp, of Buffalo, a paediatrician and an allergist who belongs to Mackarness's school, deserves to be referred to at this point. She compiled a list of typical symptoms: Hyperactive, wild, unruly-verbose (explosive, stuttering, perpetual) – inattentive, unable to maintain friendships, impulsive – short attention span – restless legs, tapping fingers – clumsy, uncoordinated, tremor – insomnia, nightmares, difficulty in falling off to sleep – nervous, irritable, indignant, sudden rage – tense, irascible, excitable – disgruntled, tired, weak, weary, exhausted, depressed, readily hurt and quick to cry – highly sensitive to smell, light, noise, pain and cold – congested or runny nose, sneezing, itchy nose – headaches, backaches, neck-pain, muscle-, joint- and growing-pains – stomach ache, nausea, digestive problems, flatulence, bad breath, burping, vomiting, diarrhoea and constipation – wetting day or night, sudden urge to pass water, burning or pain while urinating – pale, dark circles and swelling under the eyes – swollen lymph nodes in the nape of the neck – formation of fluid behind the eardrum, buzzing in the ears, dizziness – excessive perspiration – increased temperature. Some children are tired, mentally confused, irritable and depressed. Their bodies ache. They have an elevated temperature and are inclined to shiver or sweat at night. They sleep poorly, have nightmares and scream in their sleep. Other children are restless, clumsy and stutter.

They often cry and some children are cruel. They fight and have few friends. And over and over again there are problems at school!

The symptoms can be extraordinarily varied and they can even change from one hour to the next. According to Rapp this could be due to food; thus a child can be amiable but, within a few minutes of eating, he or she starts to display unacceptable behaviour.

In the early sixties Crook described fifty patients who suffered from Tension-Fatigue-Syndrome. All of them were tired, had circles under their eyes, congested noses and suffered from the symptoms described by Rapp above. Additionally, some had swollen lips – seventy-five per cent had typical, allergic symptoms, sixty-five per cent had family members who also suffered from allergies. It was always possible to recognise a trigger factor after skin testing.

Crook and his colleagues developed an elimination diet on which the patients felt well (this diet too, is very similar to ours). Thereupon systematic tests were introduced. The procedure was complicated because there were so many substances that were suspected of causing the symptoms in the patients. Presumably Crook's 'Tension-Fatigue-Syndrome' includes other illnesses besides ADD – we have been communicating with Crook and his colleagues.

Our observations show that ADD is not an allergy but a serious imbalance of the entire metabolism. It is characterised by a shift towards alkalosis, over-stimulation of the parasympathetic nervous system (an increased release of acetylcholine) and a blockage of the production of the sympathetic hormones (norepinephrine and probably dopamine), which are neurotransmitters. This imbalance indeed leads to an increased susceptibility to allergies. It triggers laryngitis in babies as one of the first allergic phenomena and later on it also includes asthma and hay fever. Almost every ADD-child had laryngitis as an infant or toddler. The imbalance begins in the mineral metabolism. Within minutes of ingesting phosphate the balance of calcium, potassium and magnesium is disrupted and the production of the neurotransmitter norepinephrine in the brain is impaired or blocked.

One cannot consider the function of norepinephrine in the brain without taking into account the fact that this same substance is the hormone of the sympathetic nervous system. ADD-children, who suffer from heart rhythm disorders and hypotonia (lack of muscle strength) to the point of collapse, evidence the profile one would logically expect to find as a consequence of this impairment of the production of norepinephrine in the brain. For this reason, when assessing a child it is not possible to understand behavioural manifestations without having precise knowledge of how they interrelate with the state of the metabolism and then it is necessary to take this into consideration. In this context we have also observed that mild stress can aggravate ADD-symptoms (cf. Wender as well) because the reaction to it rapidly increases the alkalosis. Severe stress, on the other hand, puts an end to ADD until a backlash follows.

Like Rapp, we too have observed in almost all children an obvious ghostlike pallor, with dark rings under the eyes, hypotonia with or without heart muscle disorders, a tendency to hypoglycaemia (triggered by the consumption of sugar), a tendency to eczema and a very high susceptibility to allergies. Other symptoms are: indigestion and poor growth during infancy; sleep disorders throughout all age groups – especially difficulty in falling off to sleep; furthermore a delayed twenty-four hour rhythm that makes it difficult for afflicted individuals to settle down at night and then makes it hard for them to wake up in the morning. Additionally we observed that second dentition, whose timing is determined by the activity of the thyroid gland, is frequently delayed considerably. Fifteen-year-olds who still have their baby teeth are not exceptional. As epidemiological studies attest, this late dentition is accompanied by a low susceptibility to dental caries. ADD-children are very rarely susceptible to caries. The number of children free of caries is exceptionally high. They represent more than twenty per cent of all children known to us. It is unnecessary to list every symptom again which points to impaired brain function. Equally common is the impairment in coordination between sense organs and muscles, and also between one muscle group and another. They are all exemplified in our case studies.

We were able, in a manner similar to that of Crook with his diet, to completely put an end to the entire behaviour disorder complex with all its psychosomatic symptoms by reducing phosphate intake either chemically or through diet. We were also able to cause a relapse by administering 75mg of phosphate-ions (in the form of PO_4). It is absolutely clear that phosphate-ions call forth the disorders that are described as Attention Deficit Disorder, Minimal Cerebral Dysfunction, Minimal Brain Dysfunction, Hyperactivity, etc.

The medical, psychiatric and educational approach that is being practised today will in time be merely of medical historical interest. Its methods will no longer be of practical significance. The proliferation of methods employed to treat the disorder indicates that the real cause has not yet been identified. If it can be overcome reliably by a single form of treatment, this can only mean that the real cause has been found.

2.2 THE ADD RESEARCH

The earliest and best description of Attention Deficit Disorder in childhood is 150 years old and is found in 'Struwwelpeter'[8]. The description of 'Fidgety Philip' (Zappelphilipp) is plainly that of the hyperactive, fidgety child. 'Slovenly Peter' (Struwwelpeter)[8] demonstrates total indifference to his surroundings and a high degree of

---

8: 'Struwwelpeter' is a very well-known German 19th century picture story book and was written for children in 1844 by Heinrich Hoffmann (1809 – 1894).

self-absorption. 'Frederick the Bully' (Der Böse Friedrich), who catches flies and pulls their wings off and beats up his nanny, exhibits the aggressive, cruel side of the behaviour disorder. 'Pauline the Firebug' (Paulinchen mit dem Feuerzeug) displays carelessness and thoughtlessness and, at the same time, uncontrolled compulsive behaviour (Ross and Ross: 'acts like an automaton'). 'Johnny Who Stares into Space' (Hans-Guck-in-die-Luft) lacks, as all ADD-children do, awareness and forethought, which lack leads to the relatively high incidence of accidents in ADD-children. 'Skinny Sam' (Suppen-kaspar) is the prototype of the child who is underweight, fussy and has a poor appetite. The author of 'Struwwelpeter' was a neurologist from Frankfurt; anyone who is familiar with the problems that ADD-children experience will recognise from this portrayal that a professional, sharp-sighted observer was responsible for the creation of these characters.

Scientific interest in the ADD-syndrome developed at the turn of this century which, interestingly, was when phosphate baking powder gained entry into our bakeries. In 1896 a symptom was observed in the USA which is virtually identical with the disorder known today as dyslexia (Feingold, p 18). Still described hyperactive children in 1902. He differentiated between those children with behaviour disorders who had brain lesions and those without brain damage whose intelligence was normal. He found more boys than girls suffering from "defects in moral control" and did not consider this a coincidence. He discovered boys of preschool age with uncontrollable temperaments, who scratched, bit, screamed, and who suddenly became disobedient, uncontrollable, restless, malicious and so agitated that they hit their mothers. Still thought it was conceivably a question of heredity. He emphasised the need for treatment for these children but he gave them a poor rather than a good prognosis.

Hohmann (1922), Ebaugh (1923) and Strecker and Ebaugh

(1924) observed in many of their patients who had been victims of the great epidemic of influenza encephalitis of 1918 'catastrophic personality changes', changes which did not affect the intelligence. The symptoms were very similar to those of ADD. This resemblance led to a diagnosis of brain damage even though such damage could not be proved. Not until 1935 did Childers establish that only some behaviour disorders could be attributed to brain damage. He distinguished clearly between hyperactive and brain damaged children. The first experiments to treat the syndrome with a catecholamine - Benzedrine – were made in 1935. The credit for this discovery belongs to the American Bradly. He described how patients settled down without losing their alertness. Molitch and Eccles observed an improvement in performance.

By 1950 there were about a dozen reports in existence that created surprisingly little interest. In the 1950's scientists (Strauss et al) became increasingly convinced, especially after experimenting with animals, that when behaviour changed brain damage would have to be present, even when it could not be proved. Hyperactivity was accorded special significance when it was classified as a definite indicator of brain damage. Strauss's work was highly regarded – even though it came in for a certain amount of criticism. For quite a long time it influenced attitudes towards and the handling of hyperactive children.

In 1962 a conference of the 'International Study Group on Child Neurology' was held in Oxford, England at which all those in attendance agreed to use the term 'Minimal Brain Dysfunction' (MBD) to end the controversy about damage and non-damage. This made possible the development of therapies, which would not only tinker with the symptoms but would also attempt to identify the cause.

In 1969 in Heidelberg, Germany, Müller-Kuppers, once again tackled the question – brain damage versus no brain damage. He came to the conclusion that true brain damage could be proved and would cause far greater deficits and disorders than those of ADD.

The World Health Organisation initially described ADD as Hyperkinetic Syndrome. Hyperkinetic Syndrome is but one of many symptoms. Thus one single symptom of a whole complex of symptoms was accorded a pre-eminent role which was inappropriate.

In the 1970s researchers in the USA changed their focus from the hyperkinetic syndrome to those of perception and attention[9].

Douglas and Stewart, of the University of Iowa, investigated the connection between ADD and the long term prospects for affected children from a genetic standpoint. Conners, who in the meantime had become an authority on medical and dietary methods of treatment (his questionnaires for teachers and parents are widely accepted), was especially involved in pharmaco-therapy. After this, research branched off in two different directions – on the one hand there were those who advocated psychotherapeutic methods and, on the other, those who argued for somatic causes and medical therapy. Since 1975 interest has clearly shifted towards investigating the connection with nutrition.

When we began to look into the problem of ADD, for the sake of our own son, it was still the prevalent opinion that this was a childhood illness that would end at puberty. In the meantime we have learned that ADD is a disorder whose form and effects can change but which in many cases never disappears.

Mothers first became aware of the problem behaviour of their children – the children who have been the subjects of our reports –

9: Translator's note: In the late 1970s the American Psychiatric Association defined the condition as 'Attention Deficit Disorder' (ADD) and published it in the Diagnostic and Statistical Manual of Mental Disorders (DMS III). Ten years later they included 'Hyperactivity' to the diagnosis: 'Attention Deficit Hyperactivity Disorder' (ADHD).

when their child turned two and started eating chocolate, biscuits and sausages. The children became bad-tempered, highly irritable flibbertigibbets. They shied away from being touched, were inconsiderate, 'got into everything', quarrelled with their siblings (even attacked older siblings), slept poorly, developed poorly and looked pale. At the age of three when they started attending kindergarten, they became extremely hard to handle. When the parents turned to doctors and other agencies for help, the response they often received was personal blame. In most cases these children could be rendered symptom free within a few days by reintroducing baby food and excluding milk. In this way many ADD-children can be identified quickly and precisely and thus many difficulties and much damage can be avoided.

If the condition is detected in infancy, a child's metabolism can be normalised within a few days, whereas in juveniles some conditions appear to be irreversible. But even in the case of small children the diet must be followed one hundred per cent. The 'Feingold-Association of Washington DC' pointed out in one of their information sheets the important fact that following the diet instructions even ninety per cent does not necessarily result in ninety per cent success; it results in total failure. Just as one can anticipate a chemical reaction, dietary lapses produce symptomatic relapses equally reliably.

Kindergarten teachers must be told precisely which foods the child may eat. Relapses – even in the case of small children – are caused predominantly by people who are unaware of the situation. The children themselves are only too happy to stick to the prescriptions of the diet.

The time when ADD casts a particularly dark shadow over the lives of the children is at the start of school. ADD-children are incapable of fulfilling the reasonable expectations of school but they do have the ability to disrupt the class excessively. An eight-minute report, which a head teacher prepared on a boy during class time in the fifth period of the day, makes it clear how severe the impact of inattentiveness and motor restlessness is. This 'behaviour report' is included here word for word and unabridged.

An eight-minute report:

Preliminary note – the observations were made with the approval of the class teacher by the head teacher who was seated at the back of the class where he could be seen by the students. Period of observation: – approximately eight minutes. The child was observed during the middle of the fifth lesson on a summer's day.

'Fritz' looks out the window.

Looking bored, he turns the pages of his exercise book.

Takes the exercise book and throws it for no apparent reason onto the floor, leaves it there, bends down under his desk and bites into an apple.

Before he sits up, he punches his neighbour in the ribs; the neighbour protests mildly.

Instead of responding, Fritz picks up his exercise book and puts it on the desk.

Looks at the teacher for twenty seconds.

Leans over to his bag, which is on the floor, and turns it upside down so that the contents all fall out.

Fritz fishes an adventure book out of the jumble of exercise books, sport shoes and so on and puts it on the desk, opens it at random and begins to read.

He slams the book shut.

He stands up and looks around the classroom.

When the other students look at him, he pulls faces; some laugh.

He is cautioned; he nods his head guiltily, sits down again and appears to concentrate on the lesson.

After approximately one minute he swipes the adventure book off the desk; it crashes onto the floor.

He sits quietly again.

Without warning, he punches his other neighbour.

A minor fight starts when the neighbour hits back.

Is cautioned by the teacher.

Crestfallen, he sits on his chair; pays attention.

Pulls faces again.

He pushes the scattered items on the floor together with his foot, in which process the pages in the exercise books are creased and other books are pushed into one another.

Sits up straight again and listens.

Plays vigorously with his fingers.

After being requested to put his things away, he throws them haphazardly into his bag.

He puts the adventure book in front of him on the desk, sits quietly and looks out of the window.

Suddenly, for no apparent reason, he throws the adventure book across the classroom. It hits a fellow student on the arm and falls to the floor with a bang.

The teacher loses his patience and sharply scolds Fritz.

Fritz is startled, pulls himself together.

From then on he settles down.

After reading this 'behaviour report' one can understand the despair of the teacher who is in charge of a class with a set curriculum that has to be taught to the students. The goal of the school is to educate the child. The teacher has a clear set of responsibilities; consequently the ADD-child and the school are bound to clash. It is unfortunate that educators are expected to deal with a problem, which they cannot possibly handle. It is even worse if they think they can solve the problem by using educational methods. If the functioning of the muscles of the legs – which are under conscious control – were affected in such a way as to cause lameness, it would not occur to anyone to employ educational measures. When, however, the invisible central nervous control system is affected, with the result that the ADD-child has no control over his or her muscles, the problem is considered to be an educational one. Psychotherapy can be helpful in a supplementary way but as the sole method of treatment it would be equivalent to an attempt to put out the Great Fire of London with a single bucket of water. This is even more true of educational measures – the children are 'uneducable'.

Of course a family which decides to tackle ADD with a dietary approach does not reach the 'Promised Land' for a long time. Every dietary error causes a relapse – just as predictably as hydrochloric acid and sodium hydroxide in combination turn into common salt and water. Every dietary error increases the secretion of the para-sympathetic hormone acetylcholine and blocks the release of the sympathetic hormone norepinephrine. When a child is being treated with amphetamine or Ritalin and the effect of a particular dose has worn off, violent relapses can occur. But a child can also become restless and inattentive from 11.00 am onwards at school because his or her blood-sugar level has dropped.

Teachers in particular need to understand that it is absolutely pointless to seek to deter such a child by sending home to the parents every few weeks a copy of the records in the punishment register. It would be far more constructive to send the child home or get the parents to come and collect him or her. They could then ascertain what dietary lapse had occurred. A repeat of the mistake could thus be avoided and all involved would derive maximum benefit. Parents are best advised to keep the child home for three days after a relapse. He or she is unable to learn in any case during these days – attendance would only reinforce old prejudices.

The fact that children afflicted with ADD appear to be 'nasty', arrogant, obnoxious, egocentric, disruptive, deceptive and malicious is the reason why they receive so little sympathy in kindergartens and schools. The unpopularity of these children can only be overcome by educating teachers. They must be made to understand what a battle it is for these children to achieve 'normality', as is the case with diabetics who also can only normalise their metabolism by refraining from eating many foods. This necessitates a degree of self-control in early childhood which no other child would be expected to demonstrate.

Teachers in senior high schools do not usually encounter the problem in their classes. This suggests that ADD-children all too often do not manage to reach higher levels of education. Consequently 'ADD-cases' are most evident in primary schools from year five onwards.

The picture of ADD changes in puberty. Usually a change for the worse takes place when development accelerates in pre-puberty. If development occurs in distinct spurts, the circumstances change from stage to stage. ADD can ease during the periods between growth spurts. When the gonads and ovaries finally become fully active and the sex hormones start playing a significant role in juvenile development, the prognosis is very different for males and females.

Girls once again can experience some very difficult years due to the ups and downs, which accompany the onset of maturity, during which time they are inclined to drift. The female hormones basically have the same catabolic effect on proteins as the stress hormone (epinephrine) of the adrenal gland. It counteracts the anabolic and alkaloid state of the metabolism by maintaining the equilibrium of the autonomic nervous system, thus preventing the ADD-syndrome from worsening. Just as children lose all symptoms when they have a high temperature, girls also frequently lose them when they reach full maturity. If later on in life pregnancies – which trigger another massive burst of ovarian activity – occur, the predisposition to ADD is usually eliminated. The few remaining exceptional cases are those of phosphate-sensitive women whose condition is generally due to a constitution characterised by extreme sensitivity. They must be treated and should remain on the diet.

The prognosis for males affected by ADD is very much worse because androgen markedly and considerably intensifies the syndrome. The 'awkward age' (puberty) in former times was nothing less than a sub-clinical form of ADD triggered by the male hormone androgen. This phase begins in pre-puberty during the growth spurt and is accentuated because the growth hormone and the androgens have a generalised 'anabolic' effect, causing increased protein synthesis. The greater production of protein causes increased phosphate sensitivity and is responsible for the exacerbation of the condition during puberty. Three to four vitamin B complex tablets daily will help control the activity of androgen in the liver. This on the other hand has a pronounced effect on the growth spurt in puberty. If an adolescent boy, who is going through puberty, is given his daily pH-assessment and then the right amount of diluted vinegar, his metabolism may normalise to such an extent that it will be possible to communicate with him; his verbal abilities will be restored.

The picture of post-pubertal ADD is characterised by quite typical symptoms. They are the same symptoms, which occur when the frontal lobes have been damaged: social problems and an inability to concentrate. The form of hyperactivity changes. Adolescents do not fidget any more but restlessness drives them from place to place, here and there. Typically an astonishingly high percentage of them will be found to be illiterate, not because of any lack of intelligence but due to the fact that their condition has made it impossible for them to learn to read.

These young people drift through life aimlessly. They are totally egocentric and often addicted to drugs or alcohol. In every town they have their favourite meeting places where they gather to socialise – fountains, squares, discos, pubs. Here no end of pretentious statements are made; they 'chatter senselessly'. Expressions such as 'zero-desire' and 'no-future' characterise their essential mood. Lack of motivation, which produces boredom and inner restlessness, drives them to move from place to place. This is a dangerous combination, which needs to be expressed and calls for action; it results in disputes, brawls, destruction and vandalism, and often even severe criminal offences.

In an earlier stage of civilisation symptoms disappeared between the ages of twenty-five and thirty. It was believed that the young man had 'sown his wild oats' and the unruly student had metamorphosed into a well-behaved citizen. "Gaudeamus igitur – o quae mutatio rerum" (the student's song) deplores this change as a sad event.

Kretschmer devoted a chapter of his book 'Geniale Menschen' ('Men of Genius') to the influence of turbulent hormones on human behaviour during puberty. Referring to a number of artistically creative people, he revealed that there was a pronounced blossoming of their creativity that began with puberty. He regretted that the 'splendid vitality of their youth' declined at the end of this phase, which occurred ten to fifteen years later. He described a phenomenon that affects all human beings and is particularly noticeable in artists and writers. He also referred to the fact that it was a well-known phenomenon (o quae mutatio rerum).

There are two different possibilities at the end of puberty: Either creativity simply dries up or an unruly, turbulent adolescence is replaced by a phase of maturity. Among painters working since about the turn of the century this development is evidenced by a change from dark colours suggestive of deep melancholy and depictions of gruesome, terrifying subjects to bright, sometimes even radiant colours and cheerful subjects (Cf: Kokoschka, Dix, Grosz, Van Gogh). Conversely, however, de Chirico's and Ensor's creativity stagnated and they remained stuck in a rut.

A comparable phenomenon can be observed in ADD-children

– they use dark, melancholy colours and their art work features gruesome, frightful subjects. If an end is put to ADD through diet or by purging them of excess phosphate, the dark colours and content disappear and the mood brightens. Ritalin does not have any comparable effect on their underlying mood.

One career in which an example of this change of heart is evident is that of Kubin as revealed in his autobiography and in whose life the transformation occurred at the age of twenty-five. He had experienced the characteristic, turbulent adolescence of the behaviour disturbed individual and had painted approximately six hundred 'gloomy' pictures, which he kept until his death. Around the age of twenty-five Kubin's life changed abruptly. He married and settled down and from that time on his works were scurrile and obscure, not so deeply moody as before.

It is astonishing that apart from Kretschmer nobody has taken such clear note of these rhythms or conceived of the life transformation as a fixed developmental feature. Consequently the following question has not yet been investigated: Of what significance is such a striking factor in the case of revolutionaries, or excessively aggressive people who have rigid, unrealistic goals or of cold-blooded, relentless 'agitators' (and therefore also terrorists) who likewise develop into conforming and conventional people after maturity?

The time seems ripe to research the cause of various forms of behaviour, including criminal behaviour, in a far more inter-disciplinary way than has either been done in the past or is being done today.

Only in this way can answers be found and affected individuals be provided with help in good time; i.e. before the child gets his fingers burnt.

2.3 THE EFFECTS OF PHOSPHATE IN FOOD

Chapter 2.5 will explain how phosphate comes to have an impact on the carbonic anhydrases[10]. This common impact of phosphate produces a range of consequences, which become manifest as 'illnesses' in the phosphate-sensitive person.

The general metabolism is driven towards a state of higher alkalinity – to the production of energy predominantly by oxidation reactions which, in its extreme form, results in autism (Rimland, San Diego). Dr Klemm discovered that an eight-year-old autistic child became capable of behaving like a normal child and was able to interact with other children after eating low-phosphate food. Amazingly, he also became capable of taking in most of his school lessons.

This shift towards alkalinity can be stimulated by phosphate and by acids of the citric acid cycle (such as citric or malic acids). They have a flywheel effect on oxidation reactions – energy is released and carbon dioxide levels increase dramatically, thereby stimulating the mechanism that removes carbon dioxide from the system.

Phosphate and acids of the citric acid cycle are those components in food that are responsible for the increased activity of the carbonic anhydrases. The metabolic pathway involved[11] produces acids, for example ethanol or lactate, which counteract that effect. The wide range of phosphate related disorders stems from these two conditions.

10: A zinc-based enzyme that helps regulate the acid-base equilibrium

11: It is important to understand that energy is released during cellular oxidation-reduction reactions. Cells obtain chemical energy from food molecules. This energy is converted to high-energy phosphate compounds and stored in the cells as ATP – adenosine triphosphate. An increased rate of pyruvate oxidation leads to increased ATP production.

As well as ADD, skin and sinus problems are associated with these disorders. Even babies can suffer from such allergies as cradle cap and laryngitis.

Mackarness, Randolph, Rae, Crook and Rapp claim that allergies cause the impairment of brain function. An extraordinary range of the most bizarre substances has been blamed for causing allergies but true allergens, in all cases that we came across, have been proteins of plant and animal origin.

These proteins can lead to the formation of antibodies, which make their presence felt by some form of sensitisation when they come into contact with human tissue. It is possible for a person to tolerate exposure to allergens several times, but then to respond with a full-blown allergic reaction at the next contact, a reaction that will always manifest itself through highly active amines – such as histamine. If the alkalosis in the phosphate-sensitive person can be prevented by means of vinegar or low-phosphate food, no allergic reaction will follow when he or she comes into contact with these allergens.

A five-year-old, who was allergic to all animal fibres and all pollens and had suffered from asthma as well as hay fever, became free of symptoms after he was given low-phosphate food. Four years later, when we inquired about his well-being, we learnt that he was still doing well: "Well, I'm not having any more colds", providing he kept to the diet.

An elderly woman of eighty-seven years, who had been suffering from asthma for the last fifteen years and who had been led to believe that the 'smog' in her town was responsible, had travelled to the Black Forest every winter for years because she felt considerably better there. Three years ago in summer, she began to eat low-phosphate food and since that time she has been able to stay at home in winter in spite of the 'smog' and without experiencing any severe attacks or other problems.

These examples could be supplemented by many others from the experiences of the circle of phosphate-sensitive families we are acquainted with. Asthma and hay fever in particular were symptoms that immediately responded to low-phosphate food.

From such experiences we draw the conclusion that allergies are triggered by two factors:

● By phosphate or other equally alkalising influences that act as predisposing factors and

● Once this predisposition is established, sensitisation occurs after contact with the allergens.

● If the predisposition is forestalled, contact with the allergens has no adverse effect.

The susceptibility to allergies increases with age. In women it often only emerges after menopause. When the production of oestrogen ceases, its catabolic, acidic effect also ceases. An oestrogen supplement for women after menopause becomes imperative when their oestrogen deficiency becomes evident in calcium metabolism or moodiness. Women should object if such oestrogen supplementation is denied because of the cost factor, or rather pay for it themselves (or change their doctor).

To a certain extent oestrogen provides women, even as children, with lifelong protection against the effects of phosphate. They are very much less affected by behaviour disorders than boys and men. With the onset of menopause this protection ends and phosphate begins to have a damaging effect on calcium metabolism. Calcium declines in the bones, which leads to increased bone brittleness.

In the summer of 1988 of a hundred and sixty beds in the Triemli-Hospital, Zurich, forty were occupied by patients suffering from thighbone fractures resulting from extensive osteoporosis. Before the era of antibiotics, thighbone fractures were a death sentence in most cases. The sequence of being in a plaster cast, consequently being bed-ridden and then contracting pneumonia through lack of ventilation was practically unavoidable in those days. It only became possible to pin the bones when antibiotics were introduced as a prophylaxis against infection. This shortened the period of bed-rest so much so that pneumonia ceased to be a problem. However, it is not actually necessary for calcium to decline to such an extent.

Bell and his colleagues discovered over many years of investigations in human beings and domestic animals that a single meal with a phosphate supplement could stimulate the parathyroid gland, which when activated removed calcium from the bones of young, healthy people.

When food was eaten which contained standard levels of phosphate additives, the normal daily intake of 1g phosphorus increased to 2.1g. This contradicted statements by German experts in the Federal Health Ministry, who had declared that such additives only contributed a few percentage points of all the phosphorus absorbed.

Schmidt-Gayk's study group confirmed the results obtained by Bell et al in 1986 in Heidelberg. Bell et al had merely wanted to find out what people actually consumed and in doing so they discovered that the consumption of phosphate was far too high. The consumption of phosphate in Germany was on a par with Bell's figures for the USA.

In 1963 Eichholz announced that phosphorus is a vital ingredient in our food but also that there had never been a known case of phosphate deficiency. There is a control device in the kidneys that efficiently regulates the secretion of phosphorus according to the demand for it. This secretion increases when the supply of phosphorus falls below a certain level. A phosphorous deficiency has only been observed in parenteral nourishment (drip feeding after operations) but never when a patient was eating normally. Yet the organism is sensitive to an excess of phosphorus, i.e. when a certain level is exceeded.

The allegations of three medical associations in a 1984 publication that our low-phosphate diet was a threat and would cause severe harm to health had already been proved incorrect years before their publication. These associations, furthermore, did not engage in any of their own investigative research.

It is not generally known that calcium metabolism is controlled by phosphate. To recommend milk as a prophylaxis for osteoporosis is just as absurd as recommending milk to equalise the balance of minerals. Milk contains both calcium and phosphorus in an invariable ratio but calcium metabolism is controlled solely by the phosphate blood-level. When this level increases the parathyroid hormone is activated, which triggers the removal of calcium from the bones, even if they are already deficient in calcium. A low blood-calcium level will lead to a bone metabolism disorder. A high blood-calcium level will result in calcium being deposited unevenly in the bones and also in its being deposited in inappropriate forms, such as in urinary disease as kidney-stones, in calcified scars and other forms.

The mineral content of cow's milk, from the human point of view, is unbalanced and contains an excess of phosphate. This leads to a decalcification of bone-matter and to disorders in calcium metabolism. These disorders take the form of cradle cap, gastric spasms, general indisposition and laryngitis in babies. They cease to be a problem when the children stop drinking cow's milk.

The successful treatment of calcium metabolism disorders – which include bone metabolism disorders (osteoporosis), accumulation of fluid in tissues (oedema), irritability of the nervous system and allergies – is thus only possible with low-phosphate food.

Brain activity is also affected. The exchange of neurotransmitters from cell to cell, which is brain activity in itself, requires the participation of calcium, potassium and magnesium ions.

Selye, who discovered the adrenal cortex, its function and hormones, published fourteen papers in four languages in 1958, in which he proved that phosphate, in combination with these hormones or with stress, causes severe disturbances in the potassium and magnesium metabolism. Potassium and magnesium are minerals inside the cell; sodium is an essential mineral found in tissue fluid and blood outside the cell. Muscle activity, especially that of the heart, is impaired by these disturbances. Selye succeeded in inducing the full range of heart muscle disorders with phosphate – from a simple fibrosis and a suppurative inflammation of the heart muscle to cardiac arrest. He was able to prevent these disorders by administering potassium.

The scientific community did not take any notice of these 'boring' chemical findings for twenty years, with the sole exception of a German pharmaceutical company. They put a potassium and magnesium supplement on the market. For many years this was the only available prophylactic treatment for heart rhythm disorders and other heart muscle defects.

Practically all phosphate-sensitive children and adults have potassium and magnesium deficiencies caused by phosphate excess but these disappear with low-phosphate food.

To the impairment of muscle function belong also impairments of coordination, for example of the coordination of the eye muscles. Afflicted individuals are unable to focus their eyes on one point, with rigidly parallel set pupils they stare 'unseeing' into the distance. They are not aware of anything, they cannot see or hear and one literally has to wake them.

The muscles involved in speech development are also impaired, which is why speech disorders, resulting from impaired production of sounds, are practically always associated with dyslexia. This happens so frequently that a specialised profession, that of the speech therapist, has developed to deal with the treatment of this speech disorder alone.

Difficulties with reading and writing, as well as such speech disorders, have been corrected in a large number of cases after the introduction of a low-phosphate diet. An especially aggressive five-year-old was given speech therapy for his speech disorder but when he tried the diet for four days his speech disorder and aggression disappeared. This case was so impressive that we have included this trial diet in the appendix.

Years ago we discovered the effect of phosphate on the condition of the skin. For example, a chronic, itchy eczema was driving a successful professional man to despair. When his family heard about the low-phosphate diet and strictly adhered to it, his agony – which had lasted for thirty-three years – ended four weeks later, the eczema disappeared.

Neurodermatitis is another disorder that responds favourably to low-phosphate food.

The number of people suffering from neurodermatitis has risen to more than one million in Germany alone. This complaint affects approximately 10 per cent of all babies in their first few weeks of life. Unfortunately there are no records kept on the proportion of breast– or bottle-fed children. Breast-fed babies can also be affected, as the following example of a family with four children shows:

The father had suffered from hay fever. His eldest son, aged eleven, had had behaviour problems and his other two sons, aged eight and six, had suffered from neurodermatitis. The baby, a girl, was being breast-fed and had had no symptoms – so far. This family has been on the low-phosphate diet for some time now and all members were free of complaints.

When the baby was six months old, her mother visited a close friend who tempted her with a piece of chocolate. That night the baby was very unsettled and by the following morning she had developed neurodermatitis. The mother now conscientiously keeps to the diet and the baby's neurodermatitis is in the process of healing.

Why did the baby react to the unfamiliar food in this way?

We know that all skin-ailments are linked to the breakdown of the acid mantle that coats the skin, caused by the alkalising effect of an excessive supply of phosphate.

The carbonic anhydrases initiate acid production in the stomach and the production of alkaline pancreatic juice. These secretions are adjusted, in each case, to the optimal pH-level of the digestive enzymes – gastric acid is matched to that of pepsin at pH 2.0; pancreatic juice is matched to that of chymotrypsin at pH 8.5, so that large fragments of food protein can be broken down in the acid region. Further breakdown to the amino acids then continues in the slightly alkaline region.

Clearly, disturbances to this finely tuned interplay, which are caused by phosphate, must be of great significance for the digestion on the one hand and for the regulation of the acid-base balance on the other.

It is extremely common for people with behaviour disorders to suffer also from gastrointestinal complaints and there exists a wealth of examples, such as the melancholic or the ill-humoured chronic stomach ache sufferer. These people are predominantly leptosomes (further described in chapter 2.5) who neatly fit into the category of the querulous, disgruntled, behaviour-disturbed individual. Phosphate disorders affect people from cradle to grave. They begin with the weepy baby who shies away from being touched and end with the old, osteoporotic woman, about whom the younger members of her family complain, "And my mother-in-law has become so spiteful".

Ever since we published our first observations – which point to a single cause and a principal effect – medical science has been doing its utmost to shatter the integral picture of phosphate intoxication which was presented into a plethora of individual symptoms so that it would fit neatly back into the categories of medical specialisation. A multitude of therapists are involved in treating the symptoms of phosphate-intoxication: physicians, paediatricians, allergists, psychiatrists, gastroenterologists, dermatologists, speech therapists, psychologists, physiotherapists and remedial teachers. This is a huge financial burden not only for the affected persons but also for the public health service. How easily this burden could be removed if the trouble were taken to recognise the influence of food as will be set out in Chapter 3.

2.4 EXCESS PHOSPHATE AND THE ADD SYNDROME

Aldo Massarotti, a Swiss food chemist who previously worked as Principal of the Ticino Institute of Food Control and Hygiene in Lugano, Switzerland, has described as follows the mechanisms that may explain how excess phosphate in the diet affects sensitive children and young adults:

● Phosphate diminishes the calcium concentration in the cytoplasm, which leads to an increase in alkalosis, a condition that hyperactive children frequently display. Calcium affects numerous cellular processes: it stimulates muscle contractions, controls the transmission of nerve impulses and regulates the release of neuro-transmitters. A lack of calcium ions leads to muscle cramping and pain, dyslexia due to loss of fine motor control of the eye muscles and an inability to control and coordinate muscle movement.

● Phosphate changes the calcium/phosphorus ratio, thus reducing the calcium and the magnesium concentration in the cytoplasm, which in turn leads to an alkalosis. A low level of calcium ions blocks the flow of norepinephrine and dopamine to the frontal lobes, thus leading to problem behaviour in sensitive children and young adults.

● Phosphate induces the mucous membranes to secrete

alkaline mucus. The mucous membranes normally secrete slightly acidic mucus which protects the body from being invaded by antigens and/or allergens. The allergens produce an allergic reaction and the lack of calcium, induced by an excess of phosphate, fails to prevent the antiallergenic response from occurring, which often leads to problems with asthma and other allergies.

● Phosphate inhibits intestinal absorption of calcium, magnesium, iron and zinc by forming insoluble salts in the alkaline environment of the small gut. This has a number of consequences, for example:

A magnesium deficiency impacts on those enzymes that utilize vitamin B1 to balance the nervous system and to coordinate muscle function. For this reason a calcium-magnesium supplement will help an ADD-child control his behaviour.

A lack of zinc affects the carbonic anhydrases, the enzymes responsible for maintaining the acid-base equilibrium, as described in chapter 2.5 The human system compensates by producing a metabolic alkalosis.

● Cola and other soft drinks have an undesirable effect on ADD-children, because they often contain phosphoric acid or citric acid – both being substances which ADD-children cannot tolerate – as well as caffeine and a high sugar content. (Note, however, that coffee on its own has a rather calming effect on an individual with ADD.)

● In addition to the problems described above, excess phosphate has an adverse effect on bone metabolism, because it may contribute to a condition known as nutritional secondary hyperparathyroidism. This condition may be exacerbated in individuals who consume diets rich in processed food containing phosphate additives and cola drinks, which are loaded with phosphoric acid.

2.5 WHO ARE THE ADD-CHILDREN? WHO IS AFFECTED?

Our above observations make it a reasonable assumption that the susceptibility for phosphate-sensitivity in ADD-children is inherited.

My research findings to this point in time also imply that the syndrome is inherited. Each case displays an overall similarity which is linked to personal characteristics which were defined by Ernst Kretschmer as early as 1920 ['Body Type and Character', 1980 edition]. He described three human types – leptosomes, athletes and pyknosomes. Approximately fifty per cent of the population belong to the predominant leptosome type. They can be identified by their delicate bone-structure, an elongated face, in particular a narrow lower face. A distinctive feature is pallor, which is caused by the nature of the blood circulation. Circulation is determined by the balance of osmotic pressure, the force blood exerts on the walls of the blood vessels and the pumping action of the heart. In leptosomes the pressure in the arteries is low, due to a sensitising hormone of the adrenal glands [12] which is produced by the adrenal medulla[13]. Blood pressure therefore is low, the supply of blood to the periphery is moderate and blood is inclined to pool in the abdomen. Because the supply of norepinephrine (which is released by sympathetic nerve endings and which affects overall performance) is relatively low, the parasympathetic system hormone acetylcholine [14] predominates – comparatively.

12: Also called the 'suprarenal glands'

13: The adrenal medulla produces the hormones epinephrine (adrenaline) and norepinephrine (noradrenaline) which increase the rate and force of the heartbeat.

14: Parasympathetic nerve endings release acetylcholine and sympathetic nerve endings release norepinephrine. These are chemical transmitter substances which control heartbeat, movement of involuntary muscles and the secretion of glands.

In 1931 D Jahn, a specialist in internal medicine, discovered the reason for the variation in human types. According to him there exists a range of constitutions that are based on the metabolic pathways, which enable the individual to break down carbohydrates to obtain energy during cellular respiration, and the way in which the by-product lactate (lactic acid) is removed.

In 1940 H Lampert, also a specialist in internal medicine, described the different responses to external stimuli. He combined Kretschmer's athletes and leptosomes into one group because they both respond to certain stimuli in the same way. He called them A-types to distinguish them from the pyknosome – short, stocky – B-types. Kretschmer also spoke of constitutional types but it is always a question of a range which can be placed on the Gaussian (normal) distribution curve.

Given these facts, phosphate-sensitive children can be defined precisely – they are leptosomes and athletes according to Kretschmer, A-types according to Lampert. These children predominantly gain their energy through high oxidation-reduction reactions and, according to Jahn, are provided with a so-called 'overcompensatory deacidification'. Leptosomes are characterised by reduced activity of the system that depends on hormone production by the pituitary gland[15], especially the part containing basophil cells[16]. Athletes are characterised by a predominance of the growth hormone, which is produced by the eosinophils in the anterior lobes of the pituitary gland. Growth hormones and glucagon predominate in their hormone system. In the pyknosomes, however, adrenal and gonado-trophin hormones predominate which is why they are comparatively stocky. This is a result of the early fusion of the epiphyseal cartilage (growth cartilage). They display a predominance of that part contai-

---

15: Also known as the 'hypophysis'
16: Basophils and eosinophils are white blood cells

102

ning basophils. They are not at risk to ADD.

On the other hand phosphate affects leptosomes or A-types so much that all characteristic traits are intensified and exaggerated to such an extent that the term 'healthy' is no longer appropriate to characterise the resultant condition. The disorder affects the total human being but it has its most disastrous effect on the hormone production of the autonomic nervous system. These hormones are also neurotransmitters in the central nervous system. This implies that phosphate affects the entire person but predominantly it affects the function of the newest, most highly developed part of the brain – the cerebral cortex and the frontal lobes of the cerebrum.

According to Jahn, the fundamental differences in reaction are due to variations in cellular respiration. Energy is always gained in the same way from sugar which, with the help of insulin, is brought into the cell as glucose. There in several steps the glucose is broken down into lactate, which can accumulate in the muscles and cause muscle pain and cramping. Or it can be converted via citrate (with the help of vitamin B1 as co-carboxylase) into oxaloacetate – the endproduct of this pathway. With the help of insulin, this oxalo-acetate molecule reacts with another molecule of acetyl coenzyme A (in which pantothenic acid – a member of the vitamin B complex – is contained). Thereafter it enters the so-called citric acid cycle or *Krebs cycle*[17]. Acetyl coenzyme A plays a central role in mitochondrial energy metabolism because it is the main input to the Krebs cycle. Oxaloacetate literally leaps out of the cytoplasm (where lactate is formed) into the mitochondria[18]. Thus the cell has regular

---

17: *The Krebs cycle is a metabolic pathway that involves the use of oxygen to break down glucose molecules to create energy-storing phosphate molecules.*
18: *The mitochondria are organelles that capture energy derived from food. The mitochondrial matrix is the site where the Krebs cycle occurs.*

mini organs – organelles – with functions that differ from each other. This leap of oxaloacetate from the cytoplasm into the mitochondria is normal with A-types. They have relatively high insulin activity that is responsible for this metabolic process – hence they are inclined to have a low blood sugar level and low tolerance to insulin.

In the citric-acid cycle oxaloacetate is completely broken down to carbon dioxide and water with the release of energy. In this way energy-rich molecules are created from the glucose molecule, with which the process started. During all the various stages of cellular respiration protein is broken down into amino acids. In these systems conversion to proteins is just as easily accomplished – there exist sufficient original matter and energy to synthesise protein.

The end products carbon dioxide and water are excreted. The ability of A-types to perform strenuous physical tasks is only limited by their lung capacity and their heart performance. Jahn found this among endurance athletes, for example marathon runners. Their muscles remain slim because they work extremely efficiently and it is possible to improve the performance of the lungs and the heart.

The other types are, according to Jahn, the heavyweight athletes who belong to the B-types or pyknosomes – those individuals with large muscles who predominantly obtain their energy by producing lactate. After the strain of high power performance the muscle cells are full of lactate, which either slowly continues to oxidise or is carried away in the blood stream and excreted via the liver. In this type of person the ability to perform rapidly diminishes after repeated phases of high physical effort (strain – pause – strain), whereas endurance athletes have the capacity to continue to perform at a high level for long periods.

Gaining energy predominantly through oxidation is a highly economical way of utilising food and performing physical activity.

This process affects the entire metabolism of leptosomes and their personality as well. It also leads to an acid deficiency in the system; a low level of lactate causes a deficiency of hydrogen ions. Pyknosomes, on the other hand, produce lactate under any kind of stress, which keeps the level of hydrogen ions in their metabolism consistently high.

This is a very important distinction. G. Fazekas, a Hungarian medical expert, who spent thirty-five years investigating this phenomenon, found that the hydrogen ion (of acid) has a stimulating effect on the system that depends for hormone production on the anterior lobes of the pituitary gland. He verified this in different animals. For this purpose he used simple mineral salts and was able to produce a metabolic acidosis by administering these salts as hydrogen ions. It had a lasting effect on hormone production. Fazekas could cause unmated rabbits to produce milk. Their ovaries and uteri became heavier, they contained more hormones and the adrenal glands grew bigger as well as more active. There were larger quantities of hormones in the muscles and liver and for this reason they had a more powerful influence on the entire metabolism. At the beginning of his experiments Fazekas used a variety of salts, but later used only ammonium salts because these proved to be the most consistently effective.

The gonads and the adrenal medulla are glands that synthesise sex and adrenal hormones. Specific hormones, which are secreted from the anterior lobes of the pituitary gland, stimulate the production and the release of these hormones. Consequently, the basophils in the anterior lobes of the pituitary gland must function at a relatively high level to stimulate the production of these hormones. Those individuals whose systems are highly acidic produce high levels of gonadotrophin and adrenal hormones.

Every time a baby kicks in the womb it nudges its hormonal system in a specific direction. The metabolism and the level of lactate in its blood determine which direction. This means that the development of the individual is revealed, developed and reinforced in every interaction with the environment on the basis of its genetically conditioned, inherited muscle structure. Following birth, each individual develops his personality by interacting with the environment. This can be observed in the hormonal system, the metabolism and – as we have already seen – in behaviour. His development into a unique individual, who cannot be confused with any other individual, is therefore the result of his inherited system interacting with the environment in the widest sense. Muscle activity plays a decisive role in this process because it affects the acid-base balance as well as mineral metabolism and thus influences development and performance.

Work (to sustain life), injuries, fright, fear and anger are prime phenomena. Initially they increase the level of acidity in the metabolism. The entire steady state control mechanism, i.e. the system of stress management[19], is dedicated to the removal of this acid load. This explains why the stress management system responds with increased activity and urgency every time acid accumulates in the metabolism. Accordingly it is easy to understand why a human being, who can only accomplish his or her work by producing a relatively high level of hydrogen ions (high stress level), also keeps his or her steady state control system working hard. In this way the performance of the sympathetic nervous system (which releases the norepinephrine hormone) is stabilised at a relatively high level.

It is important to understand: pyknosomes predominantly produce lactate for energy, which stimulates the sympathetic nervous system to increase its activity considerably. This in turn results in an undisturbed, stable functioning of the sympathetic nervous system

---

19: *Also called the 'steady state negative feedback control system'; it is a mechanism which is controlled and coordinated via the nervous and endocrine systems.*

and the release of norepinephrine in the frontal lobes of the cerebrum. Their brain function is not jeopardised by phosphate. Possibly, however, their serotonin system is at risk – the neurotransmitters in the limbic system which balance the moods between cheerfulness and sadness.

On the other hand, why is it so important for A-type human beings (leptosomes) to predominantly gain energy through oxidation-reduction reactions? In their system hydrogen ions, resulting from muscle activity, are few and far between. The steady state control system does not respond because it has not received a stimulus. If no hydrogen ions are produced (which are required to stimulate the steady state control system), there is no incentive for the adrenals to increase their activity to eliminate them. The steady state control system, as observed by Fazekas, does not kick into action if the glands, which depend on the basophils in the pituitary gland for hormone production are not stimulated; consequently in this situation the system will not perform at a relatively high level. Because the A-type, leptosome child develops by way of his inherited physique interacting with his immediate environment (but only in such a way as his physique allows him), the entire sympathetic, adrenal system, as well as the pituitary gland, operate on a low level. This system always runs in low gear, even at night, which in the extreme case results in a kind of endocrine 'inactivity atrophy'.

This is the person who retires from work at the age of forty-five but still has the capacity to live to a hundred years. The A-type human being is likely to reach a ripe old age without suffering from hardening of the arteries. He is not threatened – as are pyknosomes – by arteriosclerosis, diabetes, high blood pressure, etc. He is at risk though, of developing the conditions, which result from the predominance of the parasympathetic nervous system; for example gastric ulcers, tuberculosis, allergies and brain function disorders due to phosphate-sensitivity.

Several years ago an article appeared in the French weekly paper 'Le Point' that referred to Vandewalle's (from Le Pitié in Paris) findings. He had succeeded in explaining the difference in performance between endurance and power sport athletes (including short distance runners). Their capacity to perform was influenced by the different distribution of oxidising (red muscle) and lactate forming (white muscle) cells. After fifty-six years this was a morphological, anatomical verification of Jahn's physiological, chemical findings in 1931. The distribution reveals, if one does not solely consider the extremes, a normal distribution of cells. It ranges from eighty per cent white cells, which are found in the muscles of the power sport athletes (i.e. the 100m runner Ben Johnson and the downhill skier Marina Kiehl) to eighty per cent of red cells found in marathon runners. Here it is unnecessary to explain that those people, who have oxidising, red muscle cells are the ones who develop a sensitivity to phosphate and are inclined to be subject to an 'overcompensatory deacidification'. This too is a field of research that lies fallow. What influence does the so extremely divergent distribution of red and white muscle cells have, not only on muscle performance, but also on brain function and human behaviour? Kretschmer and Jahn made numerous observations on this issue but today a whole new field of research could open up from the perspective of muscle metabolism.

In a diverse population there are only limited numbers of individuals found who represent a certain extreme characteristic. The majority of people lie between the extremes. Accordingly, between the extreme of cytoplasm activity (formation of lactate) and the extreme of mitochondrial activity (the obtaining of energy by oxidation reactions), there exists a wide spectrum of people with varying degrees of phosphate sensitivity.

Gender also plays a part in determining the degree of risk. In females the hormone oestrogen displaces the response towards the B-type (pyknosomes); in males the reaction tends to go in the opposite direction. For this reason the A-type is more clearly and frequently apparent among males and consequently boys are more inclined to develop ADD. Thus protein metabolism plays an important part in the fundamental relationship between energy metabolism and personality. Anabolic proteins (male hormones) increase the tendency towards the A-type, whereas female hormones, which break down the proteins and switch them over to the formation of fat, reduce the alkalinity of the A-types and their susceptibility to the effects of phosphate.

In this way it is possible to influence the protein metabolism by switching it to anabolic or catabolic processes and therefore decreasing or increasing ADD. Gonadotrophin (sex) hormones and protein producing hormones increase ADD. Ammonium salts (which influence the amino acid metabolism of the liver in the Krebsian urea cycle by switching it to catabolic protein metabolism) are capable of transforming an ADD-child in a positive way because they stimulate the adrenal glands to release adrenal hormones.

Fazekas used ammonium chloride to give long-term relief for the symptoms of adrenal deficiency. He administered ammonium chloride tablets to his patients for three to four weeks. By imitating his methodology it proved possible to obtain equally good results with ADD.

It was a book by Jarvis that made us aware of the effect of ethanoic acid (vinegar). He had observed this in the children of apple farmers in Vermont. A teaspoon to a tablespoon of vinegar, diluted with water, has in the meantime proved its worth in countless cases worldwide. It works just as rapidly and effectively as a Ritalin tablet. It would certainly be worthwhile to investigate this correlation scientifically. How do ethanoic acid, amphetamines and the opiates balance acid/base in the human metabolism and normalise disturbed brain function? Opium derivatives inhibit cellular respiration, amphetamines release epinephrine and norepinephrine

throughout the organism and vinegar enriches the supply of H-ions.
Here, a large and not unimportant field of research lies waiting.

Carbon dioxide, which accumulates in the cells as a result of
the breakdown of glucose, is removed with the assistance of the
carbonic anhydrases. Carbon dioxide diffuses across the cell
membranes into the red blood cells where the enzyme carbonic
anhydrase converts it to bicarbonate and hydrogen ions. Carbon
dioxide is moved from the tissue to the lungs in the form of
bicarbonate and then reconverted to carbon dioxide and exhaled
from the body. But by itself, this procedure is not sufficient and
therefore kidneys, stomach, pancreas and salivary glands, all with
active carbonic anhydrases, play a role in this steady state control
mechanism, which is responsible for the individual regulation of the
acid-base balance. If, however, one of the participating systems
malfunctions, this steady state regulation will collapse. It will no
longer be possible to maintain the equilibrium or to produce
alkaline saliva – I have observed this physiologically and chemically
in a young girl with gastritis. This is a problem for the doctor and we
would become hopelessly entangled in the jungle of constitutional
causes if we attempted to influence it, without doing any good.

At present a method is resurfacing which I was able to investigate thoroughly and use thirty years ago – the determination of the
acid-base quotient according to the Frankfurt doctor Friedrich
Sander. These analyses are offered as diagnostic tools, but even
then we observed that the comparatively long drawn-out procedure
was not justified by the results it yielded. The quotients give no more
information than the simple determination of the pH-value, even
though it was most interesting to observe how, for example, the
economising of bases (OH-ions) occurred during the recovery
phase after a major, long drawn-out illness. It lasted for more than
six months, long after the afflicted person considered himself
completely recovered. For us the quotients (as described by Sander)

in correlation with the behaviour disorder are of no practical significance.

The carbonic anhydrases possess zinc as their central atom, but as yet nobody can tell us whether this element is used more, is excreted more or is absorbed more during the different stages of their activity. This too is a field of research which is currently lying fallow.

It is possible to determine a person's sensitivity to phosphate by observing the constitution of their muscles, which either produce more lactate forming or more oxidising cells, which means they have more white or more red blood cells. From all this it is also evident that the entire syndrome of the brain function disorder which is triggered by food, is both inherited and then passed on to future generations.

2.6 TARGET ORGAN – 'THE THREE PART BRAIN' (THE TRIUNE BRAIN)

In the fifties the American researcher MacLean discovered that the human brain consists of three distinct, functional, separate entities, each with its own perception, intelligence and autonomy.

The most ancient part is the brain stem, which was already developed in the saurians. Most of its functions serve to increase the chance of the survival of the individual, for self-preservation and the survival of the species. First and foremost, it controls those forms of behaviour which involve the establishment and defence of territory. Other activities include: the selection and preparation of a home site, the 'marking' of territory, self-defence, hunting, courtship and pro-creation as well as other behaviours that may be classified as guile, lying in wait and deception. As a result of imitation and habit there evolved various species, members of each of which were structurally and in their behaviour recognisable and identical, and within these species hierarchies also developed.

MacLean described the following human activities as being impulses emerging from the brain stem: obsessive compulsive behaviour; territorial defence mechanisms (keep out of my way!); pursuing 'egotistical' motives and ambitions; dishonesty, shrewdness, lies and all manner of deception; competitive behaviour; establishment of areas of influence or territories; imitating the external appearances of others; endurance and perseverance when pursuing specific goals.

According to MacLean, the brain stem is stimulated and controlled by two neurohormones: acetylcholine (the parasympathetic hormone which supplies energy; it is the workhorse of the brain) and dopamine (a forerunner of norepinephrine which regulates the brain).

MacLean also discovered a second brain and described how it encircles the brain stem. This already existed as a narrow zone in the saurians but not until the mammalian stage did it develop into an independent organ. MacLean named it the 'limbic system' – it is controlled by the indole derivative serotonin. The fluctuations in mood swings between cheerfulness and sadness, which Kretschmer considered to be characteristic of pyknosomes, originate here. Lack of serotonin is in all probability the cause of an endogenous depression, and consequently it is a metabolic disorder that develops from the metabolism of monoamines, the cause of a psychosis – a mental illness. A surplus of serotonin, on the other hand, is likely to cause alcoholism. It is assumed that it combines with acetaldehyde, the first product of the breakdown of alcohol in the liver, and that it causes alcohol addiction.

Originally the limbic system was responsible for the rearing of the helpless young and, possibly, bonding to the physical appearance of the small child (large head with chubby cheeks, plump physical shape and small limbs).

The limbic system is connected directly to the hypothalamus, the part of the brain that controls many homeostatic mechanisms[20], and which integrates body and brain and transmits information and instructions in both directions. Here, for example, information arrives from the metabolism that influences the performance of the pituitary gland, which is the gland that controls the production and release of several hormones and consequently stimulates the release of hormones from the autonomic nervous system (acetylcholine and norepinephrine).

The relationship between hypothalamus and pituitary gland is of great importance to the issue of ADD. An infuriating sight, for example, leads to a distinct increase in the activity of the sympathetic nervous system, which is related to the activation of the adrenal glands. A person flushes or becomes pale, blood pressure and pulse rate rise, the digestive activity decreases. This same auto-nomic and endocrine response, which stimulates the epinephrine-norepinephrine system, also activates the centre in the forebrain (i.e. the frontal lobes) which is responsible for moral control. Thus every emotion, which is strong enough to trigger a physical response, is simultaneously subjected to moral control. This ensures that irresponsible modes of behaviour do not occur. This system of moral supervision protects a human being from harming himself or others. It can, however, be put out of action by phosphate, alcohol, tranquillisers, fruit acid in the diet, protein-anabolic steroids, lecithin, hyperventilation – in short by the entire spectrum of those substances that inhibit that part of the brain that requires norepinephrine.

The two ancient brains are not able to express themselves in language, nor can they be reached by words. Their only means of

---

20: *Homeostasis is a control mechanism, which allows cells to carry out all their living processes by maintaining a constant internal environment despite fluctuations in the external environment.*

expression is through action. ADD children do not listen, they do not respond to reasoning, amiable requests, explanations or to threats of punishment. It is all like water off a duck's back to them – they do whatever they like. This behaviour inevitably irritates and enrages other people who do not understand why they behave as they do. It has not yet occurred to criminologists and other specialists to imagine what can happen when an overtly behaviour-disturbed child so infuriates by his non-verbal behaviour a father – who is himself affected by an on-going sensitivity to phosphate – that the father loses all self-control, which in extreme cases can lead to child abuse or even murder.

MacLean must be given credit for the discovery and definition of these non-verbal fields of behaviour. Eysenck made use of this without recognising that what he called 'extrovert' behaviour – we call it behaviour disorder – is brought about by loss of control. It is caused by the impairment of those functions that are controlled by the frontal lobes of the cerebrum. This loss of control is caused by a trigger-dose of phosphate in the phosphate-sensitive person.

The third, the most recent, the largest and for us the most important part of the brain has refined itself more and more in mammals. It has achieved its highest level of development to date in the human being. The outer layer of the brain, the cerebral cortex, transmits to us all information that arrives by way of eyes, ears and touch. It processes and coordinates, considers, thinks, remembers, forgets, makes decisions, knows and can express everything in words.

Somewhere between the Neanderthal and the Cro-Magnon era yet another change took place in human development – the frontal lobes evolved. The cerebrum expanded towards the forehead, in the direction of the eyes. This particular part of the brain is where the major damage occurs in the phosphate-sensitive person.

As we now know, nerve impulses transmit information from

cell to cell at specialised junctions called synapses[21]– this is a typical process of the entire nervous system. Chemical substances called neurotransmitters are formed and stored in the axon terminal (the nerve endings) of nerve cells in synaptic vesicles. When the nerve cell is stimulated, the neurotransmitters are released from the axon terminal where they diffuse across the synaptic cleft and bind to receptors on the postsynaptic cell[22]. This is how the central nervous system transmits information from cell to cell; it is the essence of how the nervous system functions. Which message is transmitted depends on the point at which the process takes place. In the cerebral cortex there are functional areas which have been precisely identified and which are responsible for precisely defined procedures. Thus, it has become apparent that whilst reading, visual areas in the brain are being stimulated. The neurons involved receive information, which arrives via the optic nerve. They respond by sending impulses to the eye muscles. They also process, interpret, assess and filter information. The area responsible for the movement of the speech-forming muscles is stimulated; i.e. whilst reading the eyes move to and fro – what is being seen is being converted into letters, words and meaningful sentences; a person talks silently.

The transmission of information in the cerebral cortex is dependent on the uninterrupted flow of norepinephrine between the affected cells, which is controlled by calcium and/or magnesium ions. In the ADD-child the release of norepinephrine from the

---

21: *Synapses are of two fundamentally different types: chemical and electrical, though most synapses are of the chemical type.*

22: *Fast chemical transmission takes only a few milliseconds to transmit a signal from one cell to another. Acetylcholine and glutamate are the most commonly employed neurotransmitters for fast, excitatory transmission*

synaptic vesicles is delayed or even blocked. Thus it becomes clear that the dyslexia, which so often affects ADD-children, is a result of a chemical obstruction of the area of the brain responsible for reading, which makes it futile to give remedial exercises to affected children.

Stimulants (Dexamphetamine and Ritalin) can remove the norepinephrine obstruction for a few hours. They are not able to relieve all the symptoms of ADD. Ritalin cannot brighten up the children's gloomy moods.

The effect of catecholamines on the nervous system was clarified at a major symposium in 1967. Their physiology has been understood since that time. The processes, which are controlled by the catecholamines, are affected by the information disorder of ADD. Serotonin and acetylcholine on the other hand, bind to receptors of another type.

Only recently has it been ascertained that dopamine is reduced in the cerebrospinal fluid of ADD-children. This leads to the conclusion that not only does the cerebral cortex lack conscious control, but the brain stem also lacks the ability to modulate information with the result that faulty and uncontrolled brain stem activity can constitute an additional area of breakdown in brain function.

Brain activity and the autonomic division of the peripheral nervous system are out of equilibrium in ADD-children, which cause the parasympathetic hormone acetylcholine to predominate. All the symptoms that are found in the ADD syndrome can be explained by this imbalance. Consequently ADD is a metabolic disorder relating to an imbalance of neurohormones, just as diabetes is a metabolic disorder relating to an imbalance of pancreatic hormones.

2.7 ADD AND DELINQUENCY

According to police statistics the incidence of criminal behaviour – and in particular criminal behaviour among adolescents – is rising from year to year, despite many and varied efforts and measures to prevent this. Psychiatric and psychological theories which seek to explain the causes of crime – and all suggestions for effective means of crime prevention derived from these theories – have failed all over the world.

In England, for example, an entire prison was rebuilt with small units that were easy to observe. These were managed exclusively by psychiatrists, who offered intensive psychological care. Those who were physically disadvantaged were given the opportunity to have plastic surgery. After four years, however, this prison was unable to claim any better rates of success than an old, overcrowded penal institution in Oxford. Juveniles in California who received no care returned to crime just as frequently as those who were given intensive counselling. Such results give food for thought.

Deterrence is still being attempted, although it is known that it has no effect. Criminals still receive psychological counselling, although it is to no avail. Verbal intervention does not reach those layers in the brain where criminal behaviour is established.

Science has as yet made very little impression in the field of criminology, even though it is known that chemical influences can change human behaviour beyond recognition.

Eysenck thoroughly investigated personality factors and their hereditary character. He referred to Lange's research on twins. Lange had, in addition to other studies, studied thirteen identical twins who had become criminals. The result – ten of their siblings had also committed a crime whilst three had not. In comparison, of seventeen fraternal (non-identical) twins only two of their siblings had broken the law whereas fifteen had committed no crimes during the period of investigation.

Lange conducted a study concerning seven hundred and fifty criminals, who were either an identical or a fraternal twin. He observed that the identical twin sibling had committed a criminal offence four times as frequently as the fraternal one. Eighty-five per cent of juvenile delinquent, identical twins had behaved in exactly the same way as their siblings, whereas only forty-three per cent of the non-identical twin siblings had also broken the law. In relation to homosexuality, where one identical twin was homosexual, the other was also – in one hundred per cent of cases. Among fraternal twins, on the other hand, both were homosexual in only twelve per cent of pairs. An adopted child whose natural mother had a criminal record displayed criminal behaviour considerably more often than an adopted child of non-criminal parentage. Public opinion in the USA, however, has made it difficult to accept these results, which established conclusively the influence of inherited personality on behaviour.

Public opinion has changed in the last few years since twins and triplets, who have been shown to be not only totally identical in their physical characteristics but also in their behaviour and lifestyle, have been studied. They were identical in these respects despite the fact that the children had been raised apart and were only informed of the existence of their other sibling just before the studies. The researchers who conducted the investigations admitted that they would never have believed the results had they not been their own.

These research results reduce the significance of environmental influences on human behaviour and human destiny – Eysenck still assessed it to be twenty to forty per cent – to such an extent that apart from genetic influences, food must be the most important determinant in human development. And in the diet, according to the results of our research, phosphate has the most serious influence.

Eysenck also referred to brain stem activity – as defined by MacLean – which is so important in relation to criminal behaviour, but he did not mention it in connection with the control functions of the frontal lobes. Eysenck concerned himself primarily with non-verbal functions, which he planned to influence by non-verbal mea-sures. He successfully achieved this in appropriate cases by condi-tioning patients with phobias and manias. Only incidentally did he take note of the brain chemistry. He realised that catecholamines increased the effect of the controlling influences, whereas sedatives and alcohol inhibited them. He called the former an increase of introversion and the latter was, according to him, a shift to extro-version (we consider this a loss of control in the cerebral cortex).

The term extroversion is confusing; on the one hand people with normal temperaments have the true ability to socialise; on the other, the chemically uninhibited, schizothymic, leptosomic type displays a lack of control. The former very rarely evince criminal tendencies; the latter, however, have behaviour disorders and are prone to crime. Extroversion and introversion need to be distinguished, especially since we have come to know about the phenomenon of disorders in the brain metabolism induced by food.

Eysenck also asked why people of the Enlightened (18th century) and Victorian (19th century) eras acted rationally, whereas people from later eras did not? Why was it that there was such a chasm between the biographies of artists of the Impressionist and Realist schools on the one hand and those of the Cubist, Fauvist and Surrealist schools on the other? The answer is because the food changed substantially around this time.

About 1880 sugar (with its effect of hypoglycaemia, although this was only discovered a hundred years later) became a people's food; chocolate hit the market and baking powder (half of which consists of phosphate) invaded the bakeries and kitchens.

In Chapter 2.6 (The Three Part Brain) it was explained how the organism generally controls its emotions. Eysenck observed this correlation, which is important in many ways for criminal behaviour, because it is precisely the cerebral dysfunction that allows impulses to be expressed in an uncontrolled way. And this can no longer be considered to be exclusively a problem of ADD-children, which at one stage was believed, or at least hoped to be the case. Increasing numbers of people are being found to be phosphate-sensitive even as adults. This too is a reality, which has to be factored into any concept of prevention.

All phosphate-sensitive people are to varying degrees unaware of the boundary which separates acceptable from criminal behaviour. It is a matter of chance, or rather of the prevailing circumstances, as to whether in a particular case it leads to unfortunate consequences. Athletes are especially at risk and potentially dangerous because they possess considerable physical strength.

People belonging to this category suffer from a tendency to accident-proneness, which causes them to both cause and themselves suffer many accidents (accidents involving children, traffic accidents) and which can also be regarded as verging on a form of criminal behaviour.

The impulses relating to self-preservation, procreation (sexuality), territorial defence, social hierarchy and slavish conformity to old ways of doing things (which are all controlled by the brain stem) are particularly evident in the behaviour of gangs and bands. Originally these impulses had a purpose – that of survival. Today, the threatening, martial or grotesque dress of gangs and their customary exhibitionism represent the relics, now devoid of meaning, of a formerly useful brain stem behaviour.

As we know, a strict order of rank prevails in these groups. It is absolutely clear who leads the gang and generates the violence. These rigidly led bands develop considerable criminal energies. In the meantime they have left their harmless predecessors, the Boy Scouts of yesterday, far behind.

As previously mentioned, the levels of the hormone

dopamine (the immediate forerunner of norepinephrine), which
control brain stem activity, are reduced in the cerebrospinal fluid
of ADD-children. This leads us to suspect that the norepinephrine
disorder extends to the control system of the brain stem. It would
be of immense importance to ascertain whether the control of brain
stem impulses is impaired by phosphate intoxication, as there
appear to be cases of inhumane brutality and of totally motiveless
violence in the field of crime. It can only be assumed that these
underlying impulses no longer have anything to do with the
meaningful existence and life plan of the individual, but operate
spontaneously beyond any control.

Once we have grasped the fact that the function of the frontal
lobes (which are responsible for the control of impulses from the
ancient brain) can be disrupted by phosphate intoxication, there
opens up a new perspective on criminal behaviour, especially that
behaviour which cannot be explained from a psychological point
of view.

The behaviour of an ADD-child, according to Wender, ranges
from being difficult and troublesome, through anti-social to criminal.
Behaviours, which they display in their everyday lives, are the result
of uncontrolled impulses, the impairment – to a greater or lesser
degree – of control, and 'opportunity'. How much significance each
of these particular factors has in influencing behaviour has not been
investigated as yet but the influence of each factor could be expected
to vary from individual to individual.

It is only logical to expect that behaviour occasioned by
unrestrained impulses will particularly manifest itself in contexts
where the impulse in normal circumstances would be constructive.
(Greed can be the motivation to earn an honest living through work
and effort, or it can be the motivation for illegal acquisition by means
of criminal activity).

Eysenck and Lange, as well as many others, point out the fact that since the Second World War, particularly in the last twenty years, crimes against property have increased considerably. It is primarily juveniles, whose criminal behaviours have become progressively more violent and malicious, who are responsible for these misdemeanours.

When the juvenile idealist (whose predecessor two hundred years ago was considered to be one of the most admirable 'flowers' of political and intellectual culture) degenerates and turns to primitive, violent crimes of terror; when the child of an average family is caught perpetrating a break-in in order to obtain drugs; or when bands of children from 'respectable middle class families' raid homes, summer houses or shops to take other people's belongings, simply because they want to have them – all are phenomena which cannot be explained convincingly by various moral theories, nor by 'degeneration resulting from capitalistic exploitation' nor by the constant neglect of self-centred parents. In this context, Lange placed great emphasis on the work of Frey who studied dangerous criminals and found that only a few came from criminal backgrounds. The prisoners' relatives were, as a rule, normal, peaceful and law-abiding citizens. The prisoners characterised themselves as the 'black sheep' of their families.

Even today the ADD-child is still predominantly an isolated case within the family, but the general increase in the incidence of ADD-cases can no longer be ignored. The growing sense of anxiety and personal insecurity that is spreading throughout the community is justified, in view of the unpredictability of the impulses and reactions of behaviour disturbed individuals.

The obvious parallel between the causes of ADD and criminal behaviour suggests corresponding possibilities of effective prevention – the reduction of phosphate and other associated substances (such as citric acid) in food. In the USA relevant experiments have already been undertaken. The removal of behaviour disturbing substances from the menu in American prisons (especially in 'youth detention

homes') resulted in such massive and statistically verifiable improve-
ments in the health and behaviour of the inmates, that the latter
requested the continuation of the diet. The correlation between the
consumption of milk and criminal behaviour was particularly striking
(Schauss: 'Diet, Crime and Delinquency'). In Tehama County in
California the staff in one youth detention centre suspected various
components in food, especially certain metals, as the cause of delinquent behaviour. A test, however, revealed that only one kind of food
gave rise to behaviour disorders – milk.

We too were able to observe that just a single cup of milk could
trigger behaviour disorders. Milk is a dangerous food for phosphate-
sensitive people – contrary to all conventional wisdom. This is why
milk and its derivatives must be excluded from the diet of ADD-
children until such time as an explanation is found.

The positive results of American experiments regarding nutrition and behaviour fill the pages of a book published in America
(Schauss) and in 1982 it was the topic of a symposium. The question
has to be asked: Why is this ignored by German institutions instead of
being tried out?

Once again the influence of stress, which undoubtedly can
normalise the behaviour of a person with ADD, must be emphasised.
Thus it can be observed that protest rallies escalating towards
violence dissolve when a certain level of stress is reached. The violent
individuals suddenly withdraw from the scene because they become
conscious of the consequences – self-control is now restored. Whereas for example previously they had not responded to verbal interven-
tions, attempted by the police who were trying to make them see
reason, a stress situation makes it possible for the affected person
to perceive and react normally. In such cases, stress alone offers the
chance to limit the damage. Discovery and arrest can trigger such a
level of stress in the violent individual that his or her behaviour
becomes normal for three days.

But even a criminal act itself can produce a great deal of stress. A violent criminal from Darmstadt was so shocked by his deed that he 'came to himself' and ran to the police with the exclamation, "What have I done?" This behaviour is indicative of how rapidly the warning system can be set off and how powerfully it then manifests itself.

It is of utmost importance to limit phosphate additives to a minimum in our food and in every case to list them precisely. It is simply incomprehensible that the increasing harm due to phosphate-intoxication is being thoughtlessly exacerbated as a result of legally sanctioned changes to our food. The unsuspecting, potentially phosphate-sensitive delinquent cannot avoid the harmful food and its consequences. Under these circumstances every delinquent, especially the juvenile, should have the right to have a medical assessment presented at his or her trial before the question of guilt is even discussed, particularly since it is now possible to verify the intoxication chemically. With today's level of knowledge the trite statement that the act was wilfully planned and therefore the delin-quent is responsible for his or her actions should no longer be permitted as an argument for his or her conviction. Intelligence has nothing to do with control, conscience and morality. It does not judge but serves and lets itself be used. Intelligence is no criterion for responsibility. Whether or not an individual can be held responsible for an action is a question of whether or not he is possessed of an intact, functioning conscience, of brain function which is neither poisoned nor impaired.

I can only repeat the words spoken by Adler on 31 March 1981 at the congress in the John Kennedy Clinic, John Hopkins University in Baltimore, "They are locked away even though their behaviour is beyond their own control."

In Mainz 1977, whilst eighteen year old Peter K. (a leptosomic, pale, young man) was on parole from a penal institution, he fatally injured a girl with a knife. His teacher had recorded his behavioural problems at school over a period of five years. She gave evidence as a witness at the hearing. When he was fifteen, Peter had assaulted a girl and had been sentenced to a term of imprisonment, which he had almost completed, when he again became violent while he was absent from prison. Before the fatal assault Peter had, together with his brother, drunk an excessive amount of beer and coke.

Peter was one of three sons. According to his mother, he alone resembled his father – a difficult man who often drank.

At Peter's trial, his lawyer had planned to present more detailed evidence on the behaviour disorder but the other parties involved in the case would not agree to this. The community acted as if it was the lawyer who had committed the terrible crime.

Nobody was willing to accord the delinquent the right to a thorough assessment – something we since have experienced many times because psychiatric appraisals do not consider this a criterion in their evaluations. The expert witness declared that Peter's crime was premeditated. There was nothing to suggest diminished responsibility. Despite severe behavioural abnormalities, there were considered to be no grounds for acquitting him. Consequently this eighteen-year-old delinquent was sentenced to fifteen years imprisonment. His punishment appeased the rage of the community – they felt that with the sentence justice had been done – and everybody went home satisfied.

Now, as before, Peter K. is at risk and represents a danger to the community. Phosphate and/or alcohol have the capacity to cause him to lose control at any time and thereby unleash a pattern of behaviour which has already twice caused him to offend. According to Eysenck, offenders have been known to repeat the same pattern of behaviour up to sixty times. The same is true of them as is true generally for the ADD-child – they act as if they were possessed.

With the core symptom alkalosis, which is easily accessible and measurable, research has been given a great opportunity to accurately track the shift in the metabolism. Now it is the task of criminologists and medical justice to come to terms with the implications of this knowledge. How long it will be before science takes notice will depend, among other things, on how long the victims of the intoxication continue to allow themselves to be treated and condemned in this way.

2.8 ADD AND DRUG ADDICTION

We have never doubted that behavioural problems are a halfway house on the road to drug addiction. The restlessness of ADD is a sign of extreme unease. We have so often seen it come and go and observed how moods swing in parallel with it. The restlessness and irritation are so severe that the affected individuals unanimously describe the relapses as 'terrible'. They long for nothing more than for an end to the nightmare and this is the reason why behaviour disturbed people turn to drugs.

There are four categories of substances that affect the metabolism in the same way – each produces a metabolic acidosis. These substances dispel the symptoms of ADD, but when their effect has worn off the former condition reinstates itself even more severely, depending on the affected person's level of susceptibility and his or her sensitivity to phosphate. To this group of substances belong the ammonium compounds, which can change a person's mood and which have been used for this purpose.

The same effect can be achieved with ascorbic acid but symptoms of vitamin B2 deficiency affect the skin. Catecholamines, such as Amphetamine, Ritalin and Captagon, also modify the metabolism. They can cause such ups and downs that some people on account of the relapses cannot take them.

The categories of substances that most obviously give rise to these effects are the opiates, the derivatives of morphine, i.e. heroin. Heroin instantaneously puts an end to the entire range of ADD-symptoms. It stills the restlessness and, in contrast to all the other substances, it gently and mildly lays a misty veil over the capacity to take responsibility. The world becomes blurred within a peaceful fog. 'Stoned' is the name of this condition. This is the goal, which is sought by means of heroin use: relief from restlessness and morose feelings. The intelligence is not impaired when someone takes heroin. The affected person can go about his work, may even perform well and may allow others to tell him to do this and that. Intelligence and the power of the intellect are not involved in moral consciousness, which is a separate entity.

When the effect of heroin has worn off, withdrawal symptoms manifest themselves. These cause the addiction, particularly as the withdrawal symptoms are supplemented by all the terrible emotions associated with ADD. Thus heroin has a very strong symptomatic influence on ADD and prompts an especially violent relapse.

The effect of drugs has long been known; it is only surprising that its link to the behaviour disorder has not been recognised before. This becomes clear from the fact that Catapres – a stimulant of the sympathetic nerve system – can suppress withdrawal symptoms to such an extent that drug-addicts have been known to cure themselves. It has, however, a dangerous side effect. This effect, peculiar to Catapres, is the capacity to cause a dangerous lowering of blood pressure, which in the case of drug-addicts can lead to a life-threatening situation.

In short it can be said that drug addiction can be fought only if the behaviour disorder is treated.

My practical experience in German pharmacies goes back more than fifty-five years; drug addiction, as we see it today, did not exist back then. Formerly drug addicts were sick people who received pain-killers for good reasons and who therefore had especially easy access to drugs. These were always isolated and rare cases. Consequently there must be a particular reason for the epidemic of drug addiction as well as for the crime that is so prevalent in our time.

This is one more reason to tackle behaviour disorders energetically, much more energetically than in the past. Anyone who has the care of a child in the drug milieu should give it a try.

As a result of the link between behaviour disorders, juvenile delinquency and food, Dr. Rosa Gryder of the American Food and Drug Administration predicted that the populace, the government and the economic system would come into conflict. We already have such conflict but behaviour disorders, crime and drug addiction are reason enough to use all possible means to resolve it.

To this day everything we have accomplished regarding phosphate has been achieved with the help of my husband, the kind consideration and support of some doctors, but most of all by the united efforts of parents who were just as afflicted as we were. No thanks are due to the political bureaucracies, public authorities, jurists nor in particular to medical research.

Our law-makers have done nothing for people with behaviour disturbances, for juvenile delinquents and for drug addicts – except to lock them away.

And all the time it would have been possible in each individual case, for the expenditure of less than ten dollars, in less than a week, to discover what effect phosphate was having on the phosphate-sensitive individual.

2.9 THE SYNDROME IN DETAIL – THE SYNDROME AFFECTS ALL AGE GROUPS

In 1995 we received from Switzerland the following letter (written in French): "From an early age my son Steven suffered from otitis (inflammation of the middle ear). We had a rough time as Steven never slept through the night. When he turned two, Steven went to kindergarten where his difficult behaviour attracted attention. He continually upset the dynamics of the group and created commotion among his peers. I had to deal with constant complaints from the other mothers. It was then that I observed that Steven's behaviour degenerated when he took his medication (antibiotics, cough medicine, drops, suppositories, sedatives) for his recurring otitis.

We sought advice from a naturopath who confirmed that Steven suffered from allergic reactions to milk products, pollen and other substances. She prescribed Vivigan (an antihistamine). This medication triggered a severe brain allergy. Steven lost control of his eye muscles and his limbs. He experienced amnesia and there were periods when his behaviour was autistic.

After this incident we consulted homeopathic doctors but Steven's condition continued to deteriorate. To prevent his recurring middle ear inflammations from flaring up, Steven had two operations where a drainage system was inserted in his ears. This procedure brought no relief. We suffered through the nights; the days too brought their problems. Steven developed a disturbing fascination for fire and water and created disasters with these elements. He was a danger to himself and to others. His basic mood was one of extreme dissatisfaction. Steven's behaviour was so intolerable that his presence became ever more difficult to endure. He was absolutely incapable of showing any signs of affection and over time he completely banished all harmony from our lives.

When Steven was four, two lesions appeared on his left shin and a bony deformity developed on his breastbone. His behaviour ranged from being hyperactive to being totally self-absorbed, talking incoherently and being lost in a world of his own. As well as having skin as rough as sandpaper, which erupted in places and caused intolerable itchiness, he encountered problems with his eyes. He developed a squint, which rapidly went from bad to worse.

Once again doctors subjected Steven to a myriad of tests and diagnoses, only to inform us that he suffered from the symptoms of a tumour called nodular granuloma.

Not one doctor we consulted came up with a panacea for Steven's myriad complaints (bony malformations, squint, autistic phases, hyperactivity, eczema); quite the opposite, the remedies prescribed caused more problems and eventually Steven lost the vision in his left eye.

One day, when I picked Steven up from school, I was so distressed that I was sobbing uncontrollably. One of my friends, who was a homeopathic doctor, recommended that I read a book called "La Drogue Cachée – les phosphates alimentaires" written by Hertha Hafer and translated into French by Luce Péclard. I read this book and could scarcely believe that other families had encountered similar problems. No sooner had I finished reading it, than I disposed of all products in the house with labels that listed colourings, thickeners, emulsifiers, lecithin, mineral salts, etc. On 26 October 1994 we commenced to detoxify Steven with the recommended diet. From that day on our son received food without added phosphate, according to the recommendations in the book.

We were amazed! Day by day Steven gradually metamorphosed into a normal, considerate, friendly and contented child.

As we had already made an appointment with the Hospital in Bern prior to trying the diet, we returned in November 1994 for further tests. As a result, for one week Steven had to eat the normal hospital food, despite our efforts to keep him on the low-phosphate diet. In addition, one of the tests required him to eat brewer's yeast. Twenty-four hours later Steven began to perspire profusely. His friendliness changed to bitter resentment. At night he reverted to grinding his teeth; he had nightmares; he cried and was fearful. We were right back where we had started. Steven's behaviour was obnoxious and intolerable. When Steven left the hospital, a third lesion had appeared on his shin.

At home we immediately put Steven back on the diet. Seven days later our son was once again in a good mood and able to smile.

He slept peacefully at night and behaved during the day like any other normal child. He spoke coherently and remembered things. He was no longer hyperactive. His concentration span improved tremendously; he spent long hours reading and drawing. He played harmoniously with his friends. He learned his alphabet and behaved in every which way like a child his own age. He was amicable and well-behaved at home and at school, showed an interest in his peers, and they began to enjoy his company too. He asked many questions and, naturally, he was querulous at times, just as children his age are.

There were other amazing results: The tumours reabsorbed, the recurring middle ear inflammations disappeared and Steven's vision improved with the help of spectacles. Our child has changed dramatically – he now enjoys good health and even his sinuses have been free of inflammation."

This case exemplifies how varied the syndrome can be:

1. Immunodeficiency causes the stubborn middle ear inflammation.
2. Cerebral dysfunction contributes to sudden deterioration in relationship with the social environment, but also hyperactivity which ultimately develops into autism.
3. Impairment of muscle function affects in particular the facial muscles and causes Steven to squint.
4. The lesions on Steven's shin and breastbone are clearly symptoms of poor calcium metabolism, which – in a child of Steven's age – are not the same as those of an elderly woman suffering from osteoporosis.
5. The multiple allergies lead to the conclusion that a fundamental metabolic process, which makes possible the formation of histamine, has failed. [See in this context also Pp 91-93 and 139.]
6. A shift in oxidation affects the fat metabolism, which leads

to the development of hard skin. This in turn prevents the skin from being 'lubricated' regularly. Hard fats are excreted through the skin, resulting in neuro-dermatitis.

It can be proved very readily that the full range of symptoms is triggered by our food intake, as all symptoms will disappear in the shortest time possible simply as a result of changing the diet.

We are continuously gathering ever more evidence, which casts doubt on the assumption that this syndrome is a childhood and/or an adolescence disorder. A percentage of those affected will outgrow the symptoms but many others will suffer all their lives long, right up to extreme old age. This is easily explained by the major shift in our diet, which has been developing over the last thirty years. For today the first generation of children, whom we initially observed, have long outgrown their adolescence.

This passage selected from a letter sent to us recently from the Vidar Clinic in Sweden illustrates very clearly just how severely the syndrome can affect and influence a person lifelong. It is as follows:

"We would like to bring to your attention a man who is now in his seventies. Whilst reflecting on his childhood he realised that he had suffered from a number of symptoms of the behaviour disturbed child, even though they were very mild, so that he did not have problems with them at school. He had been fidgety, had acted the fool, when teased he flew into a sudden rage and he was highly introverted. The difficulties he encountered during adolescence were probably no worse than those of others but they were not temporary as is usually the case; rather they persisted throughout his entire life. He was beginning to think that he would have to take his problems with him to the grave. It was particularly difficult for him to accept that he could not lead the contemplative, meditative life for which he was continually striving, because of his inner, strongly compulsive restlessness. All his life long he had not drunk alcohol or taken drugs – apart from phosphate, the hidden drug.

After the switch to a low-phosphate diet it took a whole six months before he was able to declare, to his great surprise, that all his problems had completely disappeared. He experienced the change as a great miracle. No less surprising was it when he suffered short but violent relapses which could, without exception, be traced back to a dietary lapse the previous day. The first time this happened he had had soybean soup and oatmeal cookies for dessert. Then twice he had gone to birthday parties and had enjoyed a piece of cake and some cookies. And finally he suffered another relapse when he was injected with a morphine-based sedative for a minor operation."

An old man, who came from a family whose members were affected by ADD and asthma, had suffered lifelong from ichthyosis – an itchy, scaly skin condition. When he moved to live with his daughter, in whose home low-phosphate food was served every day, his ailments disappeared. But one autumn when he could not resist the appeal of some delicious fruit – grapes and apples – he suffered a massive relapse and his ichthyosis returned.

On 26 July 1993 Newsweek published the results of a research program involving young adults in their mid-twenties. This program monitored the behaviour of 105 hyperactive young men and compared it to the behaviour of 100 'normal' young men. According to the report, sixteen per cent of those in the first group suffered from drug addiction and twenty-seven per cent demonstrated antisocial behaviour. In the second group three per cent suffered from drug addiction and eight per cent displayed antisocial behaviour. The young men in the first group had by this age been arrested twice as often as their contemporaries, sentenced by courts of law for serious offences five times as often and had served a term of imprisonment nine times as often.

All of this verifies the observations and experiences that we have been describing for many years.

3.0
PREVENTION

3.1 RECOGNITION OF PHOSPHATE-SENSITIVITY

To date there are no methods for curing phosphate-sensitivity but there are methods of testing to determine whether problems of the types described above can be traced to phosphate-sensitivity and are caused by food.

We recommend the four-day diet (as described in chapter five) which reintroduces plain cooking and was tested on a five-year-old boy. After three days he became entirely normal – his speech disorder and aggression disappeared. On the fifth day he drank a cup of cocoa for breakfast and with that he promptly suffered a relapse.

It is possible for a phosphate-sensitive person to normalise his or her behaviour with this four-day diet. When the symptoms have disappeared, the subject can be given a capsule of pure phosphate to provide positive confirmation of his phosphate-sensitivity. The capsules contain a mixture of 76.9mg disodium hydrogen phosphate ($Na_2HPO_4.2H_2O$) and 48.1mg potassium dihydrogen phosphate (KH_2PO_4), equivalent to 75mg PO_4. With these specifications any pharmacist could prepare such capsules.

If the symptoms are caused by phosphate-sensitivity, the subject will suffer a relapse lasting from fifteen minutes to several days. If a child responds positively to this test, it is also recommended that all members of the family be tested in the same way. This is a very reliable way of determining who is phosphate-sensitive.

PREVENTION OF PROBLEMS

There are now four known methods by which it is possible to prevent a phosphate-sensitive person from having to suffer the consequences of intoxication:

1. Methylphenidate – HCl (Ritalin) or Dexamphetamine
2. Antiphosphate (Aluminium Hydroxide or Calcium Acetate)
3. Vinegar
4. Low-phosphate food

Methylphenidate HCl is a quick acting substance but has the disadvantage of having many serious side effects. It has a symptomatic effect similar to that of a pain-killer. The administration of this medication should be restricted to those cases where it is not possible to implement the diet. Ritalin or amphetamines should not be administered over a long period of time because of their side effects. It is justifiable, however, to resort to this medication until the affected individual can recover from his or her rebellious state and follow the diet, which has the same effect as the amphetamine derivatives but without their side effects.

Antiphosphate is a purely prophylactic measure. It removes phosphate from the digestive tract before it is absorbed and thus prevents the consequences of phosphate-intoxication. It is suitable to be used when people eat in restaurants, for children's birthday parties and similar events. However, it should only be taken very occasionally.

Vinegar neutralises the alkali. It reduces the imbalance between ethanol and lactate on the one hand and maintains the equilibrium of the citric acid cycle on the other. Any kind of vinegar can be used and it is entirely irrelevant whether, or with what, it has been preserved; it stabilises the phosphate-sensitive person's condition and behaviour. Some mothers give their children vinegar diluted in water or tea to drink at school at recess and the children quickly realise that the vinegar helps them.

An objective method of monitoring the pH-value of the saliva is to measure it on an empty stomach, i.e. in the morning (prior to cleaning teeth and eating). The pH-value should be below 7.0.

The combined effect of vinegar and diet is very striking – affected children feel so much better – that it more than repays the trouble taken in the kitchen. In this way too undesirable forms of intervention, such as transferring an affected child to a special school or into a residential home for behaviour-disturbed children, can be avoided. School classes, which contain children with varying degrees of behaviour problems and a wide range of intellectual ability, make effective learning – which is the main reason for going to school – impossible.

Low-phosphate food is not a diet in the strict sense (even if the word diet is used here frequently), but food in which certain components have been reduced because persons with brain function disorders cannot tolerate them. If one makes a close study of this diet, it becomes apparent that except for milk and its by-products, it is approximately the same as the food consumed by people a hundred years ago.

Over the last twenty years, thousands of sensitive people have followed our recommended low-phosphate diet with great benefits to their well-being and without ever experiencing any health problems. There are no limits on the quantities of 'permitted' foods; it is therefore ludicrous to make assessments of malnutrition, although such assessments have been attempted. So we can continue to recommend our diet with a clear conscience as the best way to prevent phosphate-intoxication.

Low-phosphate food is therefore not a special diet that other people cannot be expected to eat. The many families, whose members have all switched to the diet after a phosphate-sensitive member led the way, confirm this among other things.

RECOMMENDED WAYS OF EMPLOYING THE
LOW-PHOSPHATE DIET

Phosphate-sensitive individuals are inclined to have a low blood sugar level, which leads to a drop in performance from 11.00 am onwards. This can be compensated for by not allowing the child to have a sweet breakfast (muesli, etc.). We recommend for breakfast: wholemeal bread and butter with salami (no additives) or a small quantity of jam. And for the mid-morning break: salami and cucumber pickles. The famous 'apple a day', to be eaten during recess, is a successful ploy of commercial agricultural promotion – in the case of phosphate-sensitive individuals, however, unsuitable because of the malic acid level.

The low-phosphate diet is also low in sugar. People very quickly adjust to the reduced intake of sugar. Fruit juices in particular have too much sugar and are loaded with malic acid, citric acid and phosphate. Sweet desserts are laden with the same acids and/or lecithin (used as an emulsifier) and cakes too belong to this category because of the eggs used.

Eggs are dangerous because the yolk contains lecithin. It is not possible to eliminate its effect with antiphosphate. The same problem applies to all soy products because they too contain lecithin.

Even though the listing of ingredients on packaged foods leaves a lot to be desired, it is still better than no listing at all. Bread bought in the supermarket, which is made of flour, water, yeast and salt and is listed as such, is quite safe. If the word 'emulsifier' is stated among the ingredients, extreme caution is essential because there is a very strong chance that this is lecithin, without it being actually so stated. This applies to all products that list 'emulsifiers' as being among their ingredients. Phosphorylated starch is also not usually listed because it is regarded as a food and not as an additive.

Of course the listing of ingredients could be as comprehensive as is the case in the USA where the influence of food on behaviour has been closely observed for approximately twenty years.

An example of an actual label is reproduced unabridged below to demonstrate to what extent the American Food and Drug Administration Authority has enforced the labelling of ingredients in packaged food:

Veal Parmigiano with Tomato Sauce

Ingredients: Minced steak: veal, beef, water, soy protein concentrate, cereals, bread crumbs, onions, sugar, salt, monosodium glutamate, seasoning, pulverised garlic.

Pastry: Water, corn flour, wheat flour, starch, salt, dextrose, acid sodium pyrophosphate, sodium bicarbonate.

Bread crumbs: Wheat flour, dextrose, sugar, salt, soy oil, paprika oleo-resin, natural aroma. The crust is coloured with paprika.

Sauce: Water, tomato paste, starch, sugar, imitation parmesan cheese with water, sodium caseinate, hydrogenated soy oil, tapioca flour, salt, tricalcium phosphate, adipic acid, artificial colouring and aroma, monosodium glutamate, potassium sorbate (preservative), cheese (parmesan and mozzarella), salt, hydrogenated vegetable protein, dehydrated onions, processed cheese with enzymes (parmesan and romano from cow's milk), flour, pulverized onions, seasoning, pulverized garlic, pulverized beetroot, citric acid, paprika, carboxymethyl cellulose, vegetable oil base (partly hydrogenated vegetable oil), lactose, sodium caseinate, dipotassium phosphate, sodium alumino silicate, butyric hydroxyanisole.

Specialists and the Federal Government[23] refuse to act unless

---

23: *Here the reference is to the German Federal Government* we can produce statistically relevant figures regarding phosphate-intoxication, conducted on a sufficiently large sample of test cases. We of course are unable to supply these data because we do not have a research facility to conduct a clinical trial. Recently in the USA, where they have had a lot more practical experience with diets, children have been taking responsibility for monitoring their own progress. This is a principle which we have employed from the outset and which we regard as correct and sensible. As an example of methodical approaches we would refer the reader to the publication, 'Disruptive Behaviour: A Dietary Approach' by Dan O'Bannion, Betty Armstrong, Ruth Ann Cummings and Judy Stange, North Texas State University. This article was published in the 'Journal of Autism and Childhood Schizophrenia' Vol. 8, No. 5, 1978, pp 325-337.

Things are so much easier for us, as we do not have to track down countless allergens or look for a global explanation, because we already have one in the phosphate-sensitivity; and due to the alkalosis, we have a definite indicator of a relapse. We believe that on this basis an investigation can be conducted as follows:

The subject's status is recorded – medical history and diagnosis. His or her disorder is remedied with vinegar and the condition that results after approximately thirty minutes is compared with the initial findings. To stabilise his or her condition, the child receives low-phosphate food, according to our directions, for a period of four to five days. Thereafter he or she is given a capsule containing 125mg phosphate buffer solution (according to Sörensen), equivalent to 75mg PO_4, pH 6.9 (cf. chapter 3). The resulting condition is then compared with the initial status. With that the test is concluded. However, the relapse which is caused by the capsule can be ended by administering vinegar. Any number of children can participate in this test, as long as their food intake is carefully monitored. This is of course so much easier than having to test every single edible item for a number of weeks for its ADD-producing effect – with the need to observe and record behaviour over a period of weeks. The observations made by O'Bannion and his colleagues are in complete agreement with ours. They noted (to my knowledge for the first time in the US literature) that the harmful effect of a food can last up to three days, which is what we have been claiming since 1975.

Psychological tests, and even more so psychiatric assessments in the field of law, have shown that current procedures of mental analysis are inadequate and misleading. There exists no statistically valid basis for comparison; there is no recognition of the extent and effect of the damage occurring in the cerebral cortex and brain stem; instead, arbitrary modes of behaviour are singled out. In comparison with themselves, however, the changes can be described objectively. This is a fact, which will eventually lead to a more realistic description of the syndrome, one that will accord with reality, especially in relation to the enormous range of ADD-symptoms – which extend from a bad mood to murderous impulsiveness on the one hand and from hypoglycaemia to an allergic crisis on the other.

Inadequate knowledge of the condition leads to people, who suffer from phosphate-intoxication, being condemned unjustly as schizoid, a condition which can not be cured by diet. There is indeed no field in society in which injustice has not been done to these people. Not even the Phosphate-League – the association we founded which has a considerable membership with the common aim of discovering a diet which will keep affected individuals free of symptoms – has to date been able to make any headway against the vested interests of so many other organisations (such as the food industry, pharmaceutical companies, Courts of Justice, schools and other educational institutions) that aim to maintain the status quo at all cost. MacLean used the terms 'defence of territory and main-tenance of power positions (will-to-power)' to characterise the reptilian brain.

3.2 LOW-PHOSPHATE FOOD IN PUBLIC INSTITUTIONS

Generally in public institutions where people of all age groups are accommodated – under duress to a greater or lesser extent or because of disadvantaged circumstances – and are catered for by communal kitchens, nothing is known about the link between food and human behaviour. Because of this lack of information, nothing is done in the field of prevention. We have not as yet had the opportunity to influence the preparation of the food in such institutions. Not even interested doctors, who would have happily introduced low-phosphate food, have been able to achieve a change.

It begins with homes for babies and culminates after children's homes, prisons and psychiatric clinics with retirement homes for senior citizens. Every phosphate-sensitive person who has to eat food from such a communal kitchen should have the right to request low-phosphate food and, if necessary, instigate legal proceedings against the institution because their physical and psychological well-being is not assured with normal food. In these institutions the inmates are often wrongly diagnosed and assessed – with far reaching consequences for their fate. Nobody recognises the 'mentally sound' person masked by the brain function disorder which is triggered by phosphate. (The possibility of remedying ADD with vinegar in a very short space of time could be put to good use in this context). Not a single person, not even qualified medical practitioners, have realised that a behaviour disturbed person first has to be given the opportunity to regain mental health before being sent for trial, a trial at which his future will be decided. The IQ of a person suffering from ADD can fall approximately twenty points below that of a person who is in full possession of his or her senses. Twenty points are equivalent to a difference between, for example, being gifted and retarded or being gifted and highly talented. Consequently, if many such people are going to be assessed and judged daily by schools and Courts of Law, methods must be employed (and to some degree they have still to be developed) such that an objective statement can be made.

Juvenile detention centres on the US West Coast achieved a forty-five per cent reduction in restless and aggressive behaviour just by eliminating soft drinks, sweets and milk. The change in behaviour was so striking that inmates and staff requested the diet be continued even after the trial period had ended. A similar result was observed in the Marl-Simsen State Hospital, which has already been mentioned above.

In the USA the savings in public expenditure per person are estimated at US$ 2,000 – 4,000 annually [24] if accommodation in a correctional institution can be prevented. These costs would be similar in Germany but no figures exist.

It is necessary to point out what effect ADD can have when it is intensified by alcohol consumption and extremist behaviour in crowd situations (which themselves have a dehumanising effect). This was demonstrated at the catastrophe, which occurred at the European Football Cup Final between Juventus Turin and Liverpool[25] in the Heysel stadium in Brussels, Belgium. Fanaticism, which can be attributed to phosphate-rich food (an English breakfast!), a susceptibility to ADD and excessive consumption of alcohol brought about a disaster in which complete abandonment of all inhibitions was reported. Furthermore, the sequence of events was precisely in keeping with the pattern of the behaviour disorder in that after the initial shock an immediate, sobering reaction occurred and the rioters came ambling meekly out of the stadium. This riot was not a 'one-of-a-kind' event – they happen worldwide. Nevertheless, a ban on alcohol is a first step in the right direction.

24: *Today these figures average US$16.000 annually per inmate.*
25: *This clash occurred on 28 May 1985 and resulted in thirty-nine deaths.*

4.0 ADVICE ON DIET AND MEDICATION

1. Follow the instructions precisely. Do not eat or buy anything that we have described as detrimental to your health or that you are uncertain about.

2. All family members should eat the same food. The phosphate-sensitive person should not be made to feel different. Furthermore, he or she will not be the only phosphate-sensitive person in the family.

3. As has been already pointed out, it is sometimes difficult to detect hidden phosphate. You can make inquiries at the head office of the large supermarket suppliers. They generally provide correct information, as they are well equipped with laboratories and usually know the precise ingredients in food.

4. The basic four-day diet, which has been included as an example of what to do, will help you get started immediately.

5. Additives in food are often listed inadequately. This will only improve if inaccurate labelling disadvantages manufacturers and suppliers. Do not buy anything if you cannot be sure what are the exact ingredients. 'Permitted additives' and similar annotations are utterly useless to our phosphate-sensitive children. We must, for instance, know precisely whether phosphate or lecithin has been used. Question the manufacturer about this and let him know that you are not satisfied with his labelling.

6. Do not worry or panic when faced with the many other substances that are added to food. For example, people have found fault with beta-carotene. This is not a poison but a colouring pigment from

carrots. The use of antioxidants in edible oils becomes more and more necessary the higher the quality of the oil. When unsaturated fatty acids become rancid, they form peroxides which are carcinogenic. As the matter stands, oil that is well preserved from oxidation is to be preferred to oil without additives.

7. The danger for our families comes from phosphate and other substances (for example milk, eggs, exotic fruit, cocoa, nuts and sugar) which have the same effect. Many foods result from agricultural overproduction or are imported from less developed countries. There is also the widespread belief that only a lack of food is harmful. People are now gradually starting to realise that it is much worse to eat to excess.

8. If, despite giving your child phosphate-reduced meals, relapses still occur, we advise strict adherence to the basic rule (e.g. the four-day diet).

Unfortunately many people blame a variety of substances (such as colouring agents, preservatives, additives and others) for causing mysterious relapses. So far no one has been able to provide positive evidence against these.

It is well worth the effort looking for hidden trigger factors (cf. Chapter 6). For example, colouring agents in chewing gum and jelly babies have been blamed as trigger agents because it was not known that chewing gum contains lecithin and jelly babies have up to one per cent citric acid.

SAFE FOOD *Eat and enjoy*	**CAUTION! DO NOT EAT,** *Will cause relapses!*

From the Bakery:

Wholemeal Bread	All other pastries
White bread, rolls and pastries if made with yeast or cream of tartar, without lecithin, milk or milk powder	All whole grains, including Ryvita
	White bread and rolls if ingredients are unknown
Shortcrust pastry, puff pastry, flaky pastry, strudel pastry and pie pastry	Frozen pastries
	Instant cake mix
Ingredients: lemon and orange peel, raisins, desiccated coconut	Commercially baked cakes and biscuits or cookies
Raising agents; sour dough, potash (potassium carbonate), sodium bicarbonate, ammonium carbonate, cream of tartar	Phosphate baking powder

Meat *Eat and enjoy*	**Meat** *Do not Eat. Will cause relapses!*
All pure fresh meat, including salted and smoked meat	Meat and sausages manufactured with phosphate additives (mineral salts, emulsifiers and lecithin)
Homemade meat broth	
Poultry and game, can be frozen	Bacon
Italian type dry sausage such as salami	Cold processed meats such as ham, bologna and other industrially prepared cold cuts
Air-dried or smoked cold cuts	Ingredients must be declared
Lard and other animal fats	Sweetbreads: kidneys, liver, brains, offal
Sausages with lactate (and listed as such), occasionally and in small quantities	Chicken or beef stock cubes
	Instant stock powder, soup mixes

Fish *Eat and enjoy*	Fish *Do not Eat. Will cause relapses!*
Fresh or frozen fish and crustaceans	Frozen fish fingers and other frozen instant fish meals
Sardines and other fish in oil	Canned fish

Eggs *Eat and enjoy*	Eggs *Do not Eat. Will cause relapses!*
Egg white – unlimited quantities	Egg yolk

Milk, Butter, Cheese *Safe Food. Eat And Enjoy!*	Milk, Butter, Cheese *Do not Eat. Will cause relapses!*
Butter – unlimited quantities	Milk – not even in small quantities, buttermilk, yoghurt
Cream – untreated fresh or sour cream	Cheese spread, all processed cheeses, cheese cake
Hard cheese in small quantities – use as a sandwich filling	Cheese dishes such as macaroni cheese, cheese soufflé, fondue and cheese bake
Cottage cheese may be spread on bread thinly	Skim milk powder, which is often added to processed foods
Homemade ice-cream using fresh cream and puréed fruit	Margarine
	Ice-cream – commercially produced

Fruit and Vegetables *Safe Food. Eat And Enjoy!*	Fruit and Vegetables *Do not Eat. Will cause relapses!*
Fresh salads and vegetables, including canned and frozen	Mushrooms
Potatoes – mash with butter and water	Sweet corn
Green peas and beans –	Soy beans and soy products (tofu, soy milk, etc.)
	Legumes – dried peas, beans,

moderate quantities

Ripe apples, pears, plums, stone-fruit – have a piece for dessert

Canned fruit, without the syrup

Jam and honey, spread thinly on bread

French fries and potato chips, homemade

Gherkin/cucumber pickles and other vegetables marinated in vinegar

lentils

Citrus fruit – oranges, lemons, limes, grapefruit

Tomatoes

Tomato paste

Puréed tomatoes

Carbohydrates *Safe Food. Eat And Enjoy!*	Carbohydrates *Do not Eat. Will cause relapses!*
Rice, semolina/cream of wheat, sago, tapioca and arrowroot	Oats, oatmeal, muesli
Durum wheat pasta	Instant rice, Instant noodles
Unbleached flour – wheat or rye	Instant pudding mixes, cold water soluble
Homemade puddings and custard – prepare with cream and water	Instant thickening such as instant gravies (i.e. cold water soluble phosphorylated starches)
Cornflour, rice flour, potato flour	Glucose, dextrose
	Pancakes
Fructose (fruit sugar)	Sugar, Honey

Beverages *Drink and Enjoy!*	Beverages *Will cause relapses!*
Mineral water	Citrus fruit drinks
Filtered tap water	Orange juice
All types of tea	Lemon juice

Freshly ground coffee	Grapefruit juice
Apple juice, cherry juice, black-currant juice, diluted with water	Fruit juices, cordial, cola, and other soft drinks
	Instant coffee
	Cocoa powder
	Milk-based energy food drinks
	Alcoholic beverages, including malt ale
Miscellaneous *Safe Food. Eat And Enjoy!*	**Miscellaneous** *Do not Eat. Will cause relapses!*
All types of vegetable oils and fats, e.g. coconut oil, copra	All types of nuts
Desiccated coconut	Almonds
Puffed rice	Nougat, marzipan
All types of herbs and spices:	Peanut butter, nut pastes
Mustard	Chestnuts and chestnut pastes
Vinegar	Popcorn
Natural flavouring essences	Yeast-paste
Pectin	Everything made from the cocoa bean, which includes chocolate
Fruit sugar	Mayonnaise
	Tomato ketchup
	Instant sauce, gravies and soup
	Instant chicken or beef stock
	Chewing gum – contains lecithin!
	Jelly babies – contain citric acid

MEDICATION

Take exceptional care with any medication. Always inform doctors and pharmacists that the patient is a phosphate-sensitive individual!

Safe Medications	Medications not to be taken *Medications can exacerbate the ADD syndrome, for example:*
Aspirin, with vitamin C Decongestant nasal drops Cough remedies, excluding codeine Tromcardin Sedatussin Calcium lactate powder	All types of sedative medicines, sleeping pills and narcotics Tranquillisers that have a sedative effect, e.g. Valium Antihistamine – has a sedative side effect, where possible replace with calcium effervescent tablets or vitamin C Energy tonics contain lecithin Frubiase-Calcium tablets contain phosphoric acid Medication containing codeine (often used in cough medicine) Antibiotics – the doctor decides whether this medication has to be administered Some medications have a high alcohol content (e.g. medicinal syrups and tinctures) Local anaesthetics that contain adrenalins Calcium Sandoz effervescent tablets.

5.0 A FOUR-DAY DIET PLAN

DAY 1

Breakfast:	Tea, bread and butter, strawberry jam
Lunch:	Tea, bread and butter, salami, cucumber pickles
Dinner:	Beef stew, vegetables, potatoes

DAY 2

Breakfast:	Tea, bread & butter, honey
Lunch:	Tea, tuna in oil, bread, cucumber pickles
Dinner:	Grilled chicken, rice (not 'instant'), salad, well-ripened fruit

DAY 3

Breakfast:	Coffee with cream, bread & butter, jam
Lunch:	Tea, bread, salami, cucumber pickles
Dinner:	Steamed fish with vegetables and potatoes

DAY 4

Breakfast:	Tea, bread and butter, jam
Lunch:	Coffee with cream or tea, bread and butter, salami, cucumber pickles
Dinner:	Rice with meat, salad, ripe fruit

The bread is a standard wholemeal loaf made from flour, water, yeast and salt.

Tea is ordinary black tea and coffee is ground from the coffee bean (not 'instant').

If additive-free salami is not obtainable substitute it for other unprocessed meats, e.g. cold roast beef or chicken.

There are no limits on the quantities of food that can be consumed.

6.0 SUMMARY

PHOSPHATE INTOXICATION

This is a homogeneous disorder that affects the endocrine and nervous systems[26] and is triggered in certain people predominantly by consuming an excessive amount of phosphate in food.

OTHER TRIGGER FACTORS

1. Sugar – especially pure glucose, fruit syrup and honey. Fructose is less harmful. Some children even transform starch into glucose so rapidly that they can suffer a relapse

2. Acids of the citric acid cycle – citric acid, malic acid, succinic acid

3. Protein anabolic substances – male hormones and progesterone derivatives (puberty!!)

4. Lecithin

5. Hyperventilation – excessive respiration of carbon dioxide and/or supply of oxygen (e.g. when playing sport or swimming in cold water)

6. Recovery phase after stress – e.g. high fever temperature, long journeys

---

26: Both are involved in controlling, coordinating and maintaining a constant state of internal balance.

CONSEQUENCES

1 Brain function disorder (affecting norepinephrine):
Hyperactivity, hypoactivity and autism
Antisocial behaviour; impulsive criminal behaviour arising from
the combination of restlessness and inactivity
   Dysfunctional muscle activity (uncontrolled movement)
   Inability of the eyes to bring an object into focus
   Dyslexia and impairment of speech
   Fear of being touched
   Inability to listen

2. METABOLISM OF MINERALS:

Calcium imbalance – leading to osteoporosis; poor healing of
bones
Irritability, cramps, pyloric spasms and laryngitis
Potassium and magnesium deficiency – resulting in poor muscle
coordination and heart muscle disorders

3. ALLERGIES:

Asthma, hay fever, urticaria, allergic eczema

4. SKIN DISORDERS:

Ichthyosis, neurodermatitis (skin that needs to be treated with
an 'acid-buffer' solution)

5. VASOMOTOR DISORDERS:

Migraines

6. GASTROINTESTINAL DISORDERS:

Stomach and duodenal ulcers

VICTIMS
WHO IS AFFECTED BY PHOSPHATE-INTOXICATION?

Phosphate affects people who were defined by Jahn in 1931 as persons who suffer from an 'overcompensatory deacidification' and who were described before that by Kretschmer as leptosomes and athletes. Their metabolism produces saliva, which is abnormally alkaline, which becomes apparent when its pH value is measured (activity of the carbonic anhydrases).

In 1987 Vandewalle, Paris, performed muscle biopsies on athletes[27] and discovered that endurance athletes have predominantly oxidising red muscle cells whereas power sport athletes have predominantly lactate forming white muscle cells. This is an extremely important indicator of personality type that is totally consistent with Jahn's findings and which demonstrates that important metabolic differences are characteristic of the same groups of athletes. Phosphate-sensitive persons are those people who predominantly have red muscle cells (leptosomes, endurance athletes).

27: *A recent (2000 report) recorded findings that about 50 per cent of marathon runners and high profile swimmers are affected by asthma. These findings are consistent with our observations.*

7.0 REFERENCES

Adler, S.J. MD, Your Overactive Child, how to help him, Insight Publishing, Los Angeles, 1980

Alabiso, F., Inhibitory Functions of Attention in Reducing Hyperactive Behaviour, Amer. J. Ment. Defic., 77:pp 250, 1972

Alexander, J., Boyle, A.J., Iseri, L.T., Caighney, R.S.LC. and Myers, Am. J. Medicine 11 p 517, 1951

Angermeier, M. (Publisher), Legasthenie, Fischer-Taschenbuch, 1977.

Arnold, Eysenck, Meli, Lexikon der Psychologie, column 1057/58, Freiburg, 1980

Bachmann, Marc R., Lebensmitteltechnologie im Kreuzfeuer der Meinung, Chimia: 42 No. 1 Januar, p 8, 1988

Bachmann, Peter, Das hyperkinetische Syndrom im Kindesalter, Hans Huber, Bern 1974.

Bachmann, Peter, Einfluss von Nahrungsphosphaten auf kindliche Verhaltensstörungen. Ein Forschungsthema in der Schweiz? Schweizerische Ärztezeitung, Bd. 68, Heft 37, 1987

Battle, E.S., Lacey, B., A Context for Hyperactive Child Syndrome, over Time: Child Development 43:pp 757, 1972

Becker, W.C., Engelmann, S., Thomas, D.R., Teaching – A Course in Applied Psychology, Science Research Associates, Chicago, 1981.

Bell, R. Rainess, Draper, H.H., Tang, F.Y.M., Shin, H.K., Schmidt, R.G., Physiological Responses of Human Adults to Foods Containing Phosphate, Additives, Journ. Nutrition, 107:pp 42, 1977

Berger, E., Minimale zerebrale Dysfunktion bei Kindern, Kritischer Literaturüberblick, Hans Huber, Bern/Stuttgart, 1977.

Birkmeyer, Walter, Die Behandlung der Depression, Der informierte Apotheker I (1974), p 24-27.

Bonting, S.L., The Effect of a Prolonged Intake of Phosphoric Acid and Citric Acid in Rats. Diss. Amsterdam, 1952.

Borbély, Alexander, Die Suche nach dem Wirkungsort von Pharmaka im Gehirn, Antrittsvorlesung a. d. med. Fakultät d. Univ. Zürich, Neue Züricher Ztg. 13.3, p 23, 1973

Bower, B.K., Mercer, C.D., Hyperactivity, Etiology and Intervention, The Journal of School Health 45:pp 195, 1975

Bradley, C., The Behavior of Children Receiving Benzedrine, American Journal of Psychiatry, 94:577-585, 1973

Brenner, A. and Wapnir, R.A., A Pyridoxine-Dependent Behavioral Disorder Unmasked by Isoniazid, Amer. Journ. Diseases of Children, 132, p 773, 1978

Bundeskriminalamt, Polizeiliche Kriminalstatistik der Bundesrepublik Deutschland, published annually, z.Zt. letztes Jahr 1982; daneben Zeitreihen von 1955 bis 1978 und 1977 bis 1981

Cane, Mc.R.A. and Widdowson, Elsie M., The Role of Inorganic Substances in the Nutrition of Aged Persons. Preisvortrag, 1970

Ausgewählte Themen über moderne Ernährung. Published by Ettore Rossi, Panscientia Verlag, Bern 1988

Childers, A.T., Hyperactivity in Children Having Behavior Disorders, Journal of Orthopsychiatry, 5:227-243, 1935

CIBA-GEIGY, Minimal Brain Dysfunction in Children, a Profile. CIBA Pharmaceutical Company, Sumnit, New Jersey, 07091. Aug. 1979

Coleman, M., et. al., Internat. Symposium on Serotonin. Ref. Selecta H. 2, p 98. 1976

Conners, Keith C., Gayette, Charles H., Southwick, Deborah H., Lees, James H. and Paul A., Androulonis, Food Additives and Hyperkineses, Pediatrics 58, pp 154-166, 1976

Crook, W.G., Harrison, W.E., Crawford, S.E. and Emerson, B.S., Systemic Manifestations Due to Allergy, Pediatrics 27:790, 1961.

Crook, W.G., The Allergic Tension-Fatigue Syndrome, Pediatrics Annals, Insight Publishing Co., New York, October 1974

Crook, W.G., Food Allergy – The great Masquerader, Pediatric Clinic of North America, pp 22: 227, 1975

Crook, W.G., Can What a Child eats make him Dull, Stupid or Hyperactive?, Journ. of Learning Disabilities, 13: 53pp, 1980

Cruickshank, W.M. (Publisher), Psychology of Exceptional Children and Youth, Englewood Cliffe, Prentice Hall, 1971

Darrow, D.C., Schwartz, R., Janicchi, J.F. and Colville, F., Journ. Clin. Investigat., 27 p 198, 1948

Declerck, A., Syndrome Hyperkinétique, Acta Paediatricia Belgica, 24, pp 587-605, cf. p 587 and p 601, 1970

Declerck, A. – quoted at – the International Study Group on Child Neurology, Syndrome Hyperkinétique, Acta Paediatrica Belgica 24:pp 587, 1970

Douglas, I.V., Sustained Attention and Impulse Control: Implications for the Handicapped Child, US-Department of Health, Education and Welfare Publ. No. (OE) 73-05000, 1974

Droese, W., Reinken, L., and Stolley, H., Phosphatzusätze zur Nahrung – Hyperkinetisches Syndrom: eine unbewiesene Behauptung, Ernährungsumschau 25:12, 1978

Dussard, Thierry, Records: Le Champion se fabrique en labo, Le Point No 781, 7. p 53, Sept. 1987

Ebaugh, F.G., Neuropsychiatric Sequelae of Acute Epidemic Encephalitis in Children, Amer. Journ. of Diseases of Children, 25: 89-97, 1923

Eichholtz, F., Riverson, E.A., Klinke, J.D., Das kalkulierte Risiko der Polyphosphate, Therapeutische Umschau Jg. XX, Heft 3, 1963

Eichsleder, W., Zur Behandlung konzentrationsgestörter, hyperaktiver Kinder mit DL-Amphetamin, Tägl. Praxis 16, pp 63-592, 1975

Euromed, H. 3, pp 106/107, Plötzlicher Kindestod. Im Schlaf. Neuere Theorien zur Aetiologie, 1974

Eysenck, H.J., Kriminalität und Persönlichkeit, Ullstein Materialien, Frankfurt 1980

Fazekas, J.G., Gewichtszunahme bei Menschen infolge Ammoniumchlorid-Behandlung, Endokrinologie 32: 289-295, 1955

Fazekas, J.G., Mästung durch Steigerung der Nebennierenfunktion, Acta. medica Szeged. Tom. XII Fasc. 2, 1949

Fazekas, J.G., Die chemischen Veränderungen des Blutes bei experimenteller Ammoniakvergiftung, Arch. f. exp. Pathol. u. Pharmakol. 180:93, 1935

Fazekas, J.G., Die Veränderungen des Blutchemismus bei exp. Laugenvergiftung, Arch. exp. Path. u. Pharmakol. 184:587, 1937

Fazekas, J.G., Die Steigerung der Nebennierenfunktion, Arch. exp. Pathol. u. Pharmakol. 198:165, 1941

Fazekas, J.G., Milcherzeugung bei virginellen Kaninchen durch Behandlung mit einfachen Verbindungen ohne Hormondarreichung, Endokrinologie 30:45, 1953

Fazekas, J.G., Experimentelle Angaben zur Beeinflussung der Ovarialfunktion, Endokrinologie 30:45, 1953

Feingold, Ben F., Why your Child is Hyperactive, Random House, New York 1974

Feinstrom, J.D., How Food Affects Your Brain, Nutrition Action 6:5-7,. Ibid. Schönthaler, St., Über den Versuch im Tidewater Detention Home, 1979

Fingerhut, M., Ruf, F. and Lang, K., Zur Frage der Resorption von Polyphosphaten, Ztschr. f. Ernährungswissenschaft, 6:288, 1966

Flade, S., Christoph-Lemcke, Ch., ARD TV-programme Ratgeber, Schule/Beruf (Bayr. Rundfunk, Red. Erziehungswissenschaften), 10.11.1980

Fleckenstein, A., Der Kalium-Natrium-Austausch als Energieprinzip in Muskel und Nerv. Springer, pp 27 Berlin 1955

Friedrich, M.H., Psychotherapeutische Verfahren in Ernst Berger: Minimale cerebrale Dysfunktion bei Kindern pp 196 Huber, Bern 1977

Glowinsky, Jaques and Baldesarini, Ross, Metabolism of Norepinephrine in the Central Nervous System, Pharmacological Reviews 18, No. 4, pp 1201. 1966

Grasser, H.H., Hafer, Hertha and Lammers, Th., Über den endogenen Schutzfactor gegen Zahnkaries in Tierversuchen an der Ratte. Ärztl. Forschung 11, p I/520-529, 1957

Gruskin, Amer. Journal of Surgery, 49:49, 1940

Hafer, Hertha, Einflüsse des Gesamtstoffwechsels auf die chemischen Eigenschaften des Speichels. Ztschr. f. prophylakt. Med. No. 3, pp 2-7, 1957

Hafer, Hertha, Über den Einfluss der Ascorbinsäure auf die menschliche Mundflora, Journ. dent. belge pp 187-198, 1959

Hafer, Hertha, Lammers, Th., Biologie der Zahnkaries, Hüthig Verlag, Energiestoffwechsel und Säure-Basen-Haushalt, pp 159-170, Heidelberg 1956

Hafer, Hertha, Diskussionsbemerkung zu Spranger in Mainzer Allg. Zeitung, 24./25.6.1978 (cf. Spranger, Prof. Dr. Interview with...).

Hafer, Hertha, Erwiderung auf Walther, B. et al in Mschr. f. Kinderheilkunde 129:56-57 (1981) mit abschliessender Bemerkung von Walther. (cf. also Walther et, al, Verändert ....).

Hafer, Hertha, Über den derzeitigen Stand des Chlorophyll-Problems, Deutsche Apothekerzeitung 96. Jg. No. 18, pp 392-394, 1956

Harbauer, H., Lempp, R., Nissen, G., Strunk, P., Lehrbuch der speziellen Kinder– und Jugendpsychiatrie, 2. edition, Springer, Berlin 1974

Harbauer, H., Einführung in die Kinder– und Jugendpsychiatrie, Ärtzte-Verlag, Cologne-Lövenich.

Hellbrügge, Th., Unser Montessori-Modell, Munich 1979

Hemminger. H.J., Kindheit als Schicksal, Hamburg 1982

Hippchen, L., Ecologic-Biochemical Approaches to Treatment of Delinquents and Criminals, Van Nostrand-Reinhild, London/ New York 1978

Hittmair, A., Wissenschaft vom Urlaub, Münchner Med. Wochenschr. 101, pp 1321-1333, 1959

Höfle, K.-H., Hyperaktive Kinder – Zu wenig Magnesium im Blut, Medical Tribune (Letter to the editor), 2. March 1979

Hohmann, L.B., Post-Encephalitic Behavior Disorders in Children, Johns Hopkins Hospital Bulletin 33:372-375, 1922

Ionescu, G., Abnormale Plasma-Katecholamin-Konzentrationen bei hyperkinetischen Kindern, Der informierte Arzt/Gazette Medicale (Basel) 17, 1665-1668, 1991

Jackson, D.D., Reunion of Identical Twins, raised apart, reveals some astonishing similarities, Smithsoniean, 11:48-56, 1980.

Jacobson, M., For the Eighties, Food and Behavior 6:3-4, No. 12/1979.

Jahn, D., Internistische Beiträge zur Kretschmerschen Konstitutions-lehre, Deutsche med. Wochenschr. 77:176-180, 1952; cf. also Arch. Klin. Medizin 170 p 26, 1931

Jarvis, D. C., 5 x 20 Jahre Leben, 29. Edition, Hallwag Verlag, Bern & Stuttgart, 1985

Kety, Seymour, Central Catecholamines in Neuropsychiatric Disorders, Pharmacologigal Reviews 18, pp 792, 1966

Kieffer, P., Spurenelemente steuern die Gesundheit, Sandoz Bulletin No. 51-53, 1979

Kindermann, W., Kritisches Alter – Die Fünfzehnjährigen, Bild der Wissenschaft 10/1981

Klöhn, E., Verhaltensstörungen – eine neue Krankheit? Mosaik-Verlag, Munich 1977

Kretschmer, E., Geniale Menschen, 5. edition, Springer, Berlin 1958

Kretschmer, E., Körperbau u. Charakter, 25. edition, Springer, Berlin 1967

Krieger, R., Zeitschr. f. Entwicklungsphysiologie und pädagog. Psychologie, H. 4, 1976, ref. Umschau 77 H.1, p 193, 1977

Kubin, A., Aus meinem Leben, DTV, Munich, 1977.

Kühne, K., Schön, R., Die Konzentrationsänderung der Elektrolyte im Plasma und im Herzmuskel unter Digitalis und ihr Einfluss auf die Digitaliswirkung, Schweiz. Med. Woschr. 1957, Beiheft zu No. 14:365.

Kühne, Petra, Reform Rundschau, 2/1987

Lampert. H., in de Rudder and Linke (ed.), Biologie der Großtadt, Steinkopff, Dresden, 1940

Landolo, C., Policlinico (Sez. Pratica), H.31, p 1146, quoted in Merckscher Monatsspiegel, 6, Heft 12, 1957

Lange, R., Das Rätsel Kriminalität, Frankfurt, 1970.

Lauersen, Fritz, Über gesundheitliche Bedenken bei der Verwendung von Phosphorsäure und primärem Phosphat in Erfrischungs- getränken, Zeitschr. Lebensmittel Unters. u. Forschg. 96:418, 1953

Lempp, R., Frühkindliche Hirnschädigung und Neurose, Huber, Bern, 1964

Lempp, R., Ursachen von Lernstörungen und ihre Bedeutung für die Entwicklung und das Verhalten der Kinder, Praxis der Psycho- therapie, XVI/1971

Lempp, Reinhart, Lernerfolg oder Schulversagen, Munich, pp 55, 1971

Lempp, Reinhart, Verhaltensstörungen im Kindesalter. 4. Verhaltens- störungen bei Schulkindern, Tägl. Praxis 17, pp 503-506. 1976

Lenhard, Hans W., Wenn Kinder Scheiben einwerfen, in der Klasse ständig stören oder sich vor Schularbeiten drücken – dann hilft keine Strafe, sondern ein Arzt. Bildzeitung, 28. Sept. 1970

Loth, Helmut, Sympathicomimetica und Sympathicolytica, Pharmazie in unserer Zeit 3, No. 2, pp 33, 1974

Löwnau, H.W., Vortrag a.d. 24. Tagung d. Nordwestf. Ges. f. Kinderheilkunde. 6.-8.6.1975, Ref. Selecta 46, pp 4264-4266, 1975

Mackarness, R., Allergie gegen Nahrungsmittel und Chemikalien, Paracelsus Verlag, 1980

MacLean, Paul, D., An Evolutionary Approach to Brain Research on Prosematic (Nonverbal) Behavior; Reprint: Labor of Brain Evolution, US Department of Health, Education and Welfare, (no year)

MacLean, Paul D., Contrasting Functions of Limbic and Neocortical Systems of the Brain and their Relevance to Psychophysiogical Aspects of Medicine, The American Journal of Medicine, Vol XXV, pp 611, 1958

MacLean, Paul D., Sensory and Perspective Factors in Emotional Functions of the Triune Brain; Reprint of the US Department of Health, Education and Welfare, NIH from Emotions – Their Parameters and Measurement, Raven Press, New York 1975

MacLean, Paul D., A Mind of three Minds, Educating the Triune Brain, 77th Yearbook of the National Society for the Study of Education, pp 308, 1978

Maickel, R.P., Cox, R.H., Ksir, C.J., Snodgrass, W.R., and Miller, F.P., Some Aspects of the behavioral Pharmacology of the Amphetamines, in Amphetamines and Related Compounds, Proc. of the Mario Negri Inst. for Pharmacological Res. Milan, Raven Press, New York 1970.

Martin, Daniel M., Hyperkinetic Behavior Disorders in Children. Clinical Results with Methylphenidate Hydrochloride, Western Medicine 8 (1967), H.1, pp 23-27.

Massarotti, A., Anomalie comportarnentali nell'età scolastica, Scuola Ticinese, N. 172, pp 7-10, Bellinzona 1991

Massarotti, A., Disturbi comportamentali – Delinquenza minorile – Alimentazione, Azione (MIGROS), Lugano October 1994

Massarotti, A., Violenza nella scuola – Alimentazione, Regione Ticino, Bellinzona March 1999.

Mergen, A., Die Kriminologie, Eine systematische Darstellung, 3. Auflage, Vahlen, Munich, 1995

Mintz, Morton, Hyperactivity in Children linked to Food Additives, The Washington Post (A9), 29.10.1973

Molitch, M., and Eccles, A.K., Effect of Benzedrine Sulfate on Intelligence Scores of Children, American Journal of Psychiatry, 94:587-590, 1937

Müller-Küppers, Manfred, Das leicht hirngeschädigte Kind, Hippokrates, pp 16/17, Stuttgart 1969

Müeller-Küppers, M., Medical Tribune, (Letter to the editor). Vasomotorische Rhinitis: Gibt's da Außenseitermittel?

Müller, Peter, Zur Wirkung von Methylphenidat bei Kindern mit erethischem Syndrom, Prax. Kinderpsycho., 20, H.2, pp 71-74, 1971

Neill, A.S., Theorie und Praxis der antiautoritären Erziehung, p 99, Rowohlt, Hamburg 1969

Oxford International Study Group, 1962. Quoted in Ben Feingold: Why your Child is Hyperactive, p 18 Random House, New York, 1974

Petzet, Heinr. W., Kubin, A., Kartograph des Schattenreiches, Weltkunst, H.9, p 925, 1977

Pichotka, J., von Kügelgen, B., and Damann, R., Die Bedeutung der Schilddrüse für die Temperaturregulation, Arch. exp. Path. Pharmakol. 220, 398, 1953

Pirlet, K., Die Lampert'sche Reaktionstypenlehre in ihrer Bedeutung f. d. Ärztl. Praxis, Der Landarzt 28, H.14, pp 1-11, 1952

Pontius, A., and Walker, N.K., Rep. No. 63 Amer. Psychiatr. Ass. Ann. Conf. Miami May 1976: Electronic Test Data (ZITA/EDT) compared with the hypothesis that 85% of MBD is a Frontal Lobe System Dysfunction.

Poustka, F., Schwarzbauh, H., Eisert, H.G., in: Ernst Berger, Minimale cerebrale Dysfunktion bei Kindern, pp 169-196, Huber, Bern 1977

Rapp, D. Allergies and the Hyperactive Child, Cornerstone Library, Simon and Schuster, New York 1976

Ross, D.M. and Ross, Sh.M., Hyperactivity – Research, Theory and Action, John Wilex and Sons, New York 1976

Schauss, A.G., Behaviour Problems and Biochemicals, Science News, April 1981

Schauss, A.G., Diet, Crime and Delinquency, Parker House, Berkeley/California 1983

Schmidt, M.H., Das hyperkinetische Syndrom im Kindesalter, Zeitschrift für Kinder- und Jugendpsychiatrie, Bd. I, 3:250-270, 1973

Schmidt, M.H., Behandlung des hyperkinetischen Syndroms bei Kindern unter Berücksichtigung von Ätiologie und Pathogenese, Pädiatr. Praxis, 14:205-214, 1974

Schmidt, M.H., Verhaltensstörungen bei sehr hoher Intelligenz. Huber, Bern 1977

Schmidt-Gayk, H., Kohlmeier, M., Hitzler, W., Der Phosphatbedarf des Menschen, Akt. Ernähr. II (1986), pp 142-144.

Schönthaler, St., cf. Feinstrom.

Seelig, M.S., Vitamin D and Cardiovascular, Renal and Brain Damage in Infancy and Childhood, Annals of the New York Acad. of Sciences Vol. 147, Art. 15, pp 537-582.

Selbach, H., Fortschritte der Neurologie, 17:129 and 151 (1949) quoted in Frowein and Harrer, Vegetativ endokrine Diagnostik, Urban u. Schwarzenberg, p 12, Berlin 1957

Selecta 1974: No. 47, pp 4222, Biologische Aspekte der Schizophrenie. Lectures from the Science Writer's Seminar on a Biological View of Mental Illness, New York 3. May 1974

Selye, Hans, Experimental Production of Endomyocardial Fibrosis, pp 1351-1353, The Lancet 1958

Selye, H., Humoral Conditioning for Production of Acute Massive Myocardial Necroses by Neuromuscular Exertion, Proc. Soc. Exp. Biol. Med. 96 pp 512-514, 1957

Selye, H., Erzeugung der Phosphat-Steroid-Kardiopathie durch verschiedene Steroid-Hormon-Derivate, Ztschr. f. Kreislaufforsch. 47, pp 318-326, 1958

Selye, H., Prevention of the Phosphate-Steroid-Cardiopathy by Various Electrolytes, American Heart Journ. 55, pp 163-173, 1958

Selye, H., Humoral Conditioning for the Production of a Suppurative Acute Myocarditis by the Oral Administration of Sodium Phosphate, Amer. Heart Journ. 55 (1958), pp 1-7.

Selye, H., Nonspecifity of the Mechanism that Elicits Myocardial Necroses in Humorally Conditioned Rats, Endocrinology 62 (1958), pp 541-543.

Selye, H., The Humoral Production of Cardial Infarcts, Brit. Med. Journ. 1 (1958), pp 599-603.

Selye, H., Synergism between Mineralo- and Glucocorticoids in the Production of the Phosphate-Steroid-Cardiopathy, Acta Endocrinologica 28 III, pp 279-282, 1958

Selye, H., On the Site of Interaction between Na H_2 PO_4 and $MgCl_2$ or K Cl in the Prevention of the Phosphate-Steroid Cardiopathy, Acta Endocrinologia 28, pp 273-278. III, 1958

Selye, H., and Renaud, Serge, Prévention par la chlorure de potassium d'une myocardite purulente expérimentale, La Presse médicale 66, pp 99-101, 1958

Shaywitz, S.E., Cohen, D.J., Shaywitz, B.A., Biochemische Basis der Minimal Brain Dysfunction, The Journal of Pediatrics 92: pp 179, 1978

Silbergeld, E.K., Goldbey, A.M., Lead-induced behavioral dysfunction: Animal Model of Hyperactivity, Exper. Neurol. 42, pp 146-157, quoted in 39a, 1974

Sinz, D., Neuentdeckt, Léon Spillaert, ein Außenseiter gewinnt an Bedeutung, Artis 33:H. 12, p 37, 1981

Smith, Lendon, Feed Your Kids Right, Mac Graw Hill, 1979

Sommer, Erika, Diktat Note 6, Klett Verlag, Stuttgart 1973

Spranger, Prof. Dr., Interview mit..., Normalkost macht viele Kinder krank, and: Phosphatarme Diät ist umstritten, Mainzer Allgem. Zeitung vom 4.6.1978. Diskussionsbemerkung dazu von Hafer, H., ibid. 24./25.6.1978

Still, G.F., The Coulstonian Lectures on Some Abnormal Physical Conditions in Children, Lancet, 1:1008-1012, 1077-1082, 1163-1168, 1902

Stolley, H., Kersting, M., Droese, W., and Reinken, L., Bemerkungen zu einer sogenannten phosphatarmen Diät für Kinder mit hyperkinetischem Syndrom, Mschr. f. Kinderheilkunde, 127:pp 450 (cf. Droese), 1979

Strauss, A.A. and Kephart N.C., Psychopathology and Education of the Brain-injured Child, Vol. II. Progress in Theory and Clinic. Grune and Stratton, New York 1955

Strecker, E.A., and Ebaugh, F., Neuropsychiatric Sequelae of Cerebral Trauma in Children, Archives of Neurology and Psychiatry, 12:433-453, 1924

Tower, D., (NIH Bethesda), 13, Kongress der Intern. Liga gegen Epilepsie in Amsterdam, Ref. Euromed. No. 2, p 144, 1978

Ungerstedt, Urban, Stereotaxic Mapping of the Monoamine Pathways in the Rat Brain quoted in Borbély, Acta physiologica Scandinav., Suppl 376, pp 1-48, 1971

Van Genderen, H., Report on the Activities of the National Institute of Public Health in the Netherlands in the Field of Food Additives. (1949-1955) quoted Phosphat-Symposion 1956, Ludwigshafen,

Benkkiser, Ludwigshafen, 1956, p 93; Van Genderen, H., Die Pharmakologie der kondensierten Phosphate im Zusammenhang mit der Anwendung dieser Stoffe als Lebensmittelzusätze, ibid., pp 147-157.

Van Genderen, H., Phosphatbedarf und Grenzen der Phosphatzufuhr, Ztschr. f. Ernährungswissenschaft, Suppl. I, pp 32-43, 1961

Walther, B., Dieterich, E., Spranger, J., Verändert Nahrungsphosphat neurophysiologische Funktionen und Verhaltensmerkmale hyperkinetischer und impulsiver Kinder?, Mschr. f. Kinderheilkunde 128: 382-385 (1980) (cf. Hafer, H., Erwiderung...).

Weiss, G. and Hechtmann, L., The Hyperactive Child Syndrome, Science Vol 2. 205:28, 1979

Wender, P.J., Minimal Dysfunction in Children, John Wilex and Sons, New York 1971

Whalen, C. and Henker, B., (publisher), Hyperactive Children. The Social Ecology of Identification and Treatment, Academic Press inc., London 1980

Winter, Peter, Der Einsame am 'Ball der toten Ratten'. 'du', Europäische Kunstzeitschrift, Zurich March 1978

Various Reports, Essays and Newspaper Articles:

'Zappeln bezwungen', Der Spiegel, 9.11.1970

Hot Dogs and Hyperkinesis, Newsweek, 9.7.1977

'Fehl am Platz' Der Spiegel No. 45/1975

Wenn die Schrift aussieht wie Drahtverhau, Heptner, Frankf. Allgemeine Zeitung 10.12.1975

Hilfe für bewegungsgestörte Kinder, Mainzer Allgem. Zeitung
4.5.1977

Elfjähriger Junge erstach Schwester, Mainzer Allgem. Zeitung
4.5.1977

Frauen im Untergrund, Etwas Irrationales, Der Spiegel, 8.7.1977

Phosphatarme Diät ist noch umstritten, Interview mit Prof. Spranger,
Mainzer Allgem. Zeitung, 10.6.1978

Berichte über die Ernährungsversuche des Jugendamtes in
Rückersdorf, Nürnberger Zeitung and Nürnberger Nachrichten
from 25. March to 10. April 1979

Normalkost macht viele Kinder krank, Mainzer Allgem. Zeitung,
4.6.1979

Unruhigen Kindern kann geholfen werden, Zeitschrift 'Eltern',
January 1981

Mit Fünfzig aus Gesundheitsgründen pensioniert... Neue Züricher
Zeitung, 6.6.1981